THE FAMILY

P. M. ABBEY & E. M. PAULSON-BOX

THE FAMILY

Illustrations by Moira Büj

METHUEN EDUCATIONAL

LONDON · SYDNEY · TORONTO · AUCKLAND

First published in Great Britain 1982
by Methuen Educational Ltd
11 New Fetter Lane, London EC4P 4EE
Copyright © 1982 P. M. Abbey and E. M. Paulson-Box
Printed in Great Britain by
Richard Clay (The Chaucer Press) Ltd, Bungay, Suffolk

ISBN 0 423 50890 3

Miss Abbey was formerly principal lecturer
at the F. L. Calder College of Education.
Mrs Paulson-Box is lecturer in Home Economics
at the F. L. Calder College of Education.

By the same author
'*O' Level Cookery* P. M. Abbey and G. M. Macdonald
(Methuen Educational 4th Ed. 1976)

ACKNOWLEDGMENTS

The authors wish to express their gratitude to:

Mrs E. Anderton, Librarian at F. L. Calder College, for her invaluable assistance with reference material.

Mr B. Lawless for checking the text on Health.

Mr E. A. Paulson-Box for checking the text concerned with Physics and Chemistry.

Mrs B. M. Rayworth for typing assistance.

Merseyside Police for permission to reproduce the leaflet on page 47 and the Controller of Her Majesty's Stationery Office for permission to reproduce part of an income tax form on page 80.

CONTENTS

INTRODUCTION

The family is the nucleus of a community and is responsible to a great degree for the happiness and well-being of its members. Because societies are composed of families, improvements in family life should benefit communities, both national and international. A family consists of individuals who are bound together in a unit but who need to be considered in their own right. This book provides information about family members from the unborn child to the elderly person, and considers health, food and clothing, and finance.

In the past, families usually had to be self-sufficient. There was little provision by a government for health care. Until well into the twentieth century in the United Kingdom, diphtheria, tuberculosis and many other diseases were quite common. At the present time, in many parts of the world, disease is endemic. It has been stated that one child in ten dies before the age of five years. In 1959 the United Nations adopted the Declaration of the Rights of the Child. Principle 4 states:

> *The child shall enjoy the benefits of social security. He shall be entitled to grow and develop in health; to this end special care and protection shall be provided both to him and to his mother, including adequate prenatal and postnatal care. The child shall have the right to adequate nutrition, housing, recreation and medical services.*

As an individual grows, care and protection should continue to try to ensure that people lead healthy and contented lives into old age.

Food is an important factor in health. A knowledge of the nutritional needs of individual family members should help to provide a balanced diet. However, many people do not have a basic knowledge of nutrition, and food technology has developed a wide variety of foods. These factors, together with the pressures of advertising, may make it difficult for wise nutritional provision. While malnutrition occurs in some affluent societies, undernutrition is causing the death of many people in the world.

The clothing needs of a family are important. Since the Second World War, textile technology has developed a great variety of fibres and fabrics. A knowledge of family needs and consumer rights should enable value for money.

The welfare of a family and of individuals is much dependent upon finance. In the United Kingdom, a system of state financial provision did not really function until the middle of the twentieth century. Although this provision is now adequate, it is necessary for people to take responsibility for financial matters.

Conditions in society which affect people change, as technology develops new materials and methods, and there is research into health care. People need information and guidance to adapt themselves to changing conditions and to resolve the different problems met in the various stages of life. Information provided by a course of study in Home Economics should aid this adaptation.

REFERENCES

Text and illustrations on domestic and social history:

Domestic Life in England Norah Lofts (Weidenfeld & Nicholson)
Victorian Lancashire Ed. S. Peter Bell (David & Charles)
Victorian and Edwardian Liverpool and the North West from old photographs (Batsford)
Our Daily Bread: Food and standards of living – the fourteenth century to the present day R. Thames (Penguin)

Fiction of the period:

Oliver Twist Charles Dickens
Her Benny Silas K. Hocking
The Water Babies Charles Kingsley

FOLLOW-UP ACTIVITIES

1. Visit libraries; museums.
2. Talk to old people.
3. Research into social and domestic conditions in the nineteenth and beginning of the twentieth centuries.
4. Consider the changes in household equipment and materials over the last century.

USE OF THE BOOK AND DEVELOPMENT OF COURSES

This book has a modular structure. A module is perceived as a unit of information and study which is complete in itself but can contribute to a sectional field of study, e.g. the Baby and Child Care Module is a course in its own right, but could be combined with other modules to form a sectional study of The Family.

Using the book, it is possible to develop courses which vary in depth and duration according to pupil needs. Course planning is aided if a curriculum development approach is implemented.

The following curriculum model, which has been used as a basis for the planning of the modules, is suggested:

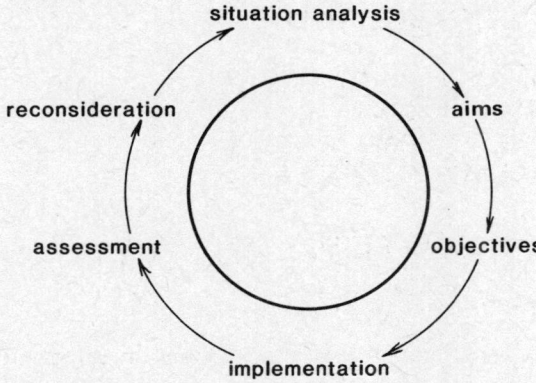

Aims are listed.

Objectives for each module are provided at the end of the book. A study of the module should enable achievement of the objectives.

Follow-up activities are suggested at the end of each module.

References which are provided at the end of each module will need updating at intervals. Developments in science and technology obviously have a considerable impact on the study of Home Economics. Knowledge should be updated by consulting current sources of information.

THE FAMILY

AIMS

To develop an awareness of the roles of family members.

To foster a knowledge of child development.

To consider factors contributing to positive health.

To examine family finance and consumer education.

IDENTIFICATION OF THE FAMILY

A family is a small group who choose to live together in one household and take responsibility for rearing their children. Family life in this country tends to follow a pattern: a man and a woman set up home together and probably produce and rear children, who usually leave and set up homes of their own. In turn they produce and rear children. The grandparents now live as a basic family again. This pattern is described as the family life cycle. In the stages of this cycle, the individuals play different roles – a man as a son, brother, uncle, husband, father, grandfather; a woman as daughter, sister, aunt, wife, mother, grandmother.

TYPES OF FAMILIES

THE BASIC FAMILY

This is the first stage of the family life cycle – a couple who together have not produced children.

THE NUCLEAR FAMILY

Parents and children live together in one household. An elderly relative may also reside with the family.

THE SYMMETRICAL FAMILY

The traditional roles of husband/father and wife/mother merge and responsibilities and tasks are shared/exchanged, e.g. a woman may go out to work and a man may work at home.

THE SINGLE PARENT FAMILY

Reasons for this type of family:

a) *Death*
One parent has died and the other is left with the responsibility for the children. There may be problems of a practical, financial and emotional nature.

b) *Separation or divorce*
This is increasingly common. There may well be problems as in (a) above and possibly more insecurity for the children and an effect on their relationships with others.

c) *Decision not to marry*
A woman may decide to bring up her children without the ties of a marriage.

d) *Employment taking one parent away from home*
Seamen, members of the armed forces and people working abroad are in this category. The responsibilities of the remaining parent are considerable.

THE EXTENDED FAMILY

This term refers to a broad family structure made up of small family units held together by kinship. It includes parents, unmarried children and married children, their spouses and children. Contact between members may be regular or confined to family occasions such as weddings, christenings or funerals.

THE EXPERIMENTAL FAMILY

Examples are the Kibbutzim in Israel or societies/communes which may have a religious basis.

FUNCTIONS OF THE FAMILY

a) *Provision of residence and security*
A residence is necessary for stable home life. Without it, the other functions are difficult to fulfil satisfactorily. Family members have certain

basic material and psychological needs which can only be fulfilled successfully within the security of a home.

b) *Co-operation*
This is needed to carry out the work of the household and for the effective management of money and resources.

c) *Reproduction*
Without this function, society would cease to exist and so it is valued. In some cultures a woman has to prove her fertility before being allowed to marry.

d) *Socialisation*
In this process the child should learn from adults the knowledge, skills and attitudes for life in the family and in the community.

e) *Relaxation*
The pressures of everyday living cause stress. The family is able to provide support and comfort so that the individual can face physical and emotional challenges. There will probably be an increasing amount of leisure time in the future, therefore it is important that there are activities in which families can participate.

DEATH IN THE FAMILY

A death in the family causes shock and distress. At the same time certain arrangements and legal responsibilities have to be undertaken. By law, the death must be registered at the district office of the Registrar of Births and Deaths. Death certificates will be issued which are required for funeral arrangements, and by the DHSS (Department of Health and Social Security), insurance companies, and for other matters concerned with the Estate of the deceased. Domestic and financial matters will need attention. Advice may be obtained from the Citizens Advice Bureau or from the DHSS.

SUMMARY

It is essential to appreciate that while patterns of family life vary according to culture, the family is universal and there is no adequate substitute. Without stable family life, societies world-wide and nationally could be adversely affected.

MODULE ONE   REFERENCES

The Family M. Waddington (Batsford)
The Family Richard Cootes (Longman)
Domestic Life in England N. Lofts (Weidenfeld & Nicholson)

FOLLOW-UP ACTIVITIES

1. Consider the role you play in your family in relation to other family members.
2. Write a short paragraph about:
   a) A nuclear family
   b) An extended family
3. Find out about family structures in other countries by consulting a library and talking to people from other parts of the world.
4. Find out about family life in the nineteenth century.

BABY AND CHILD DEVELOPMENT

PARENTHOOD

Becoming a parent involves major changes and adjustments in the life style of a basic family. There will be a change in the relationship between the man and the woman, both during pregnancy and especially after the arrival of the new baby. There can be changes in economic circumstances if the decision is taken by one parent to stay at home and look after the baby. The quality of antenatal and postnatal care received is vital for the health and development of the baby and the health and well-being of both parents.

CONCEPTION

Every month, in a healthy, menstruating female one ripe egg (ovum) matures and is released from one of the ovaries. This release of the ovum is called ovulation and it usually occurs 14 days before the start of the next menstrual cycle. The egg travels towards the womb (uterus) down the fallopian tube where, if there are sperms present, fertilisation (conception) occurs. During sexual intercourse the male's penis is inserted into the female's vagina. On ejaculation about 500 million tadpole-shaped sperms are released in 3–4 cc of seminal fluid. Only a few hundred sperms complete their journey to the fallopian tubes. If intercourse occurs during the female's fertile period, then only one of the millions of sperms released may succeed in fertilising the ovum. Sperms live for about 36 hours and probably take approximately 6 hours to swim to the site of fertilisation. The fertilised ovum proceeds down the fallopian tube and becomes implanted in the wall of the uterus. Conception has occurred and except for any adverse developments, this will result in a term of pregnancy (normally 9 months) and the birth of a baby.

SIGNS OF PREGNANCY

a) missed period;
b) short scanty period;
c) changes in breasts: heavy, tingling, darkening around nipples;
d) need to urinate more frequently;
e) constipation;
f) nausea (not necessarily only in the morning – can be throughout the day);
g) changing tastes: may be metallic taste in mouth; reaction against coffee, tea, highly seasoned foods;
h) increased vaginal discharge;
i) being more tired than usual;
j) if a smoker, feeling a decreasing need for a cigarette.

These signs are common to other illnesses but if sexual intercourse has occurred *without* contraceptive precautions being taken, conception could have occurred. It is then vital to seek professional advice which usually results in a pregnancy test.

TESTS TO CONFIRM PREGNANCY

Usually done on a urine sample.

Can be done by, general practitioner, family planning clinic, British Pregnancy Advisory Service, chemist, commercial agency. ('Do-it-yourself' kits are available but not recommended.)

If pregnancy is confirmed, the doctor will issue a 'certificate of expected confinement' showing the expected date of birth. This certificate is necessary to claim State benefits: free prescriptions during pregnancy, maternity grant, maternity allowance, free dental treatment until the child is one year old.

ANTENATAL CARE

It is important for the health of the baby and mother to have a pregnancy confirmed as early as possible. Late confirmation and delay in attending, or not attending, the clinic can cause increased risks, even death, to both mother and child. Twenty-five per cent of pregnant women in Britain do not report for their first antenatal visit until well into pregnancy. Attendance at antenatal clinics is not just for first-time parents and it is advisable for the father to attend for at least one visit.

The antenatal clinic may be held at a doctor's surgery, a Health Centre, in the hospital where the birth is to occur, at a National Childbirth Trust session.

On the first visit

a) confirmation examination;
b) mother is weighed – advisable not to put on more than 10 kg during pregnancy;
c) urine sample to check for diabetes, albumin, pus;
d) blood pressure;
e) blood test to check:
   i) blood group.
   ii) haemoglobin level – anaemia.
   iii) for venereal disease.
   iv) for other diseases, especially if mother born abroad;
f) discuss medical history of both parents;
g) check size and position of baby;
h) calculate or confirm expected week of confinement – date of last normal period will be required for this;
i) note father's job;
j) note living accommodation.

Subsequent visits

At 4-weekly intervals until 28 weeks.
At 2-weekly intervals from 20 to 36 weeks.
At 1-week intervals from 37 weeks until labour begins.

If the mother's health causes concern, visits may be more frequent. Tests b, c, d, e(ii) and g (see above) are repeated each visit. Other tests may be carried out to try to detect abnormalities. If the mother is unsure of any details concerning pregnancy, clinic attendance or birth, she should not be afraid to ask. It is useful to write down problems as they occur so that questions can be asked at subsequent visits.

CARE PROCEDURE

The advice of the doctor must be followed.
a) *Diet – (Refer 'O' Level Cookery or a nutrition book).*
b) *Clothing*
    1. Choose loose fitting, comfortable clothing in minimum-care fabrics.
    2. Underwear should give correct support to breasts and back.
    3. Special tights give support to legs carrying extra weight and decrease risk of varicose veins.
    4. Shoes should have heels of medium height and be well fitting, comfortable and able to support weight correctly.
(Refer Module 10)

c) *Rest, relaxation, exercise and fresh air* – all are essential. Pregnancy is not an illness but it does put a strain on the mother's body. The best advice is to rest when tired; some mothers need more rest than others. Try to ensure 8 hours sleep is taken at night. When resting, put the feet up if possible. Exercise is beneficial in moderation in a normal pregnancy. Correct posture is important.

d) *Recreation* – leisure activities are important. If possible some leisure time should be shared with the baby's father so that he feels involved.

e) *Personal Hygiene* – particular care should be given to personal hygiene, special attention paid to breasts if intending to breast feed. Care of teeth and gums is important, but there is no evidence to confirm the theory that the baby takes calcium from the mother's teeth if her diet is deficient. (*Refer Module 6*)

f) *Sex* – there is no reason why this should not continue if it is the wish of both partners and the pregnancy is normal. Consult the doctor if in doubt.

g) *Drugs* – most dangerous during the first 3 months of pregnancy, when greatest foetal development occurs. If pregnancy is being considered and the mother is taking any drugs, the doctor should be consulted. No drugs or medicines, not even pain killers, should be taken without the permission of the doctor. It is especially important never to take drugs prescribed for someone else. (*Refer Module 6*)

h) *Alcohol* – can effect foetal development. (*Refer Module 6*)

i) *Smoking* – can affect the growth of the developing foetus and the future baby. Mothers who smoke:
    1. Have an increased risk of miscarriage.
    2. May have smaller babies.

3. Increase the risk of perinatal death.
4. Can cause their children to have an increased risk of respiratory diseases and infections.
5. Cause a decrease in the amount of oxygen being transported to the baby across the placenta.
6. Transmit fewer nutrients to the baby across the placenta.

('Passive' smoking can also affect the baby since the mother is inhaling in a smoky atmosphere.) Consult the doctor and take his advice. (*Refer Module 6*)

PREGNANCY

1. Seven days after conception the fertilised ovum has become a ball of cells – the outer layer of cells becomes the placenta, which acts as the life-support system for the baby, the inner cells develop into the baby over the next 39 weeks.

2. During the second week, the inner cells begin the development of:
a) skin, brain, eyes, ears and teeth;
b) the amniotic sac which is filled with fluid in which the baby floats;
c) the lungs and the digestive tract.

3. In the third week another layer of cells begins the development of:
a) the heart, blood, muscle, kidneys;
b) the umbilical cord which connects the baby to the placenta.

The placenta transmits nutrients and oxygen; removes carbon dioxide and waste products; protects from illness and some drugs; produces some hormones.

4. By the fourth week the embryo should have developed:
a) a recognisable head and limb buds;
b) sites (places) for the eyes;
c) a heart beat.

5. At the eighth week the baby is recognisably human and is called a foetus. It is about 25 mm long. All the main organs of the body are formed but not fully developed.

6. At the twelfth week the skeleton and muscles have developed and there is co-ordination of the brain and the other organs. But the foetus is only 75 mm long and too small to survive outside the uterus. It is possible to identify the sex from the heart beat and because the external genitals appear.

7. During the 4–6 month period the mother's abdomen begins to bulge

as the foetus grows rapidly in the watery environment of the amniotic fluid. The foetus is exercising limbs, practising breathing, swallowing, passing urine, hearing and seeing.

8. In the 7–9 month period foetal growth continues as layers of fat are laid down under the skin. At 28 weeks the foetus is called a baby and survival outside the uterus is possible. By the end of the pregnancy the head has moved down into the lower part of the uterus in preparation for birth.

BIRTH

Indications that the birth is about to occur are spots of blood, the waters breaking and contractions.

The birth is divided into three stages – labour, delivery, afterbirth.

During labour

The cervix is gradually widened (dilated) by the contractions of the uterine wall muscles.

At the end of this stage the baby's head should be seen and the mother should have an urge to push downwards with each contraction.

During delivery

a) the birth of the head occurs, usually face downwards;
b) the eyes and mouth may need cleaning;
c) the head should rotate and the rest of the body emerge;
d) outside air must enter the lungs; this may occur naturally or be induced. At this stage, generally, the baby cries;
e) the umbilical cord is clamped and cut;
f) the baby is examined, weighed and measured and returned to the mother, hopefully in the father's presence.

During the afterbirth

The placenta separates from the uterine wall in a final contraction.

Some babies are born in the breech position (feet first); or by caesarian section; or with the aid of forceps.

Various methods of pain relief are available during labour, but some mothers prefer a natural birth.

THE PLACE OF BIRTH – HOME OR HOSPITAL?

This decision must be taken early in the pregnancy. It is advisable to have the baby in hospital if the mother:
a) is under 17 years and over 35 years;
b) is having her first or fifth subsequent baby;
c) has health problems during pregnancy which have given cause for alarm;
d) is diabetic;
e) has a small pelvis and a caesarian is contemplated;
f) is having a multiple pregnancy;
g) has home circumstances which are not suitable – poor facilities, over-crowding, and some distance from a hospital;
h) has a history of miscarriages;
i) has rhesus negative blood;
j) has had one baby already by caesarian section;
k) has vaginal bleeding before labour.

BIRTH REGISTRATION

By law (Births and Deaths Registration Act 1953) it is the duty of:
a) the father/mother; or
b) another qualified person (in the case of the death or inability of the father/mother) who was either
   (i) the occupier of the house in which the child was born, or
   (ii) present at the birth, or
   (iii) in charge of the child,
to register the birth of the child at the office of the Registrar of Births and Deaths in the sub-district in which the child was born. Registration must take place within 42 days from the date of birth or a fine will be imposed. If circumstances prevent registration, the Registrar should be contacted.

POSTNATAL CARE

Six weeks after a normal birth the general practitioner will carry out a postnatal examination. If it has been a difficult birth, this should be carried out at the hospital where the baby was born.

The doctor will give an internal examination to ensure that the uterus is back in place; check progress with feeding; ascertain the state of health of the mother and baby, and give contraceptive advice.

The mother is recommended exercises which should help her to regain her figure and to keep fit and healthy.

BABY'S FIRST MEDICAL EXAMINATION

This is necessary to check that the baby is normal and healthy; if this is not so, treatment can be started without delay. Usually the medical occurs during the first 24 hours after the birth. Obvious severe abnormalities will usually have been attended to immediately after the birth.

MEDICAL PERSONNEL CONCERNED WITH PREGNANCY

a) *General Practitioner*
b) *Midwife*
   A state registered nurse who has taken additional training and qualifications concerned with the delivery of babies and their immediate postnatal care. May be a member of the hospital staff or the Primary Health Care Team.
c) *Health Visitor*
   An experienced state registered nurse, with midwifery training, who has taken further studies in community nursing.
d) *Obstetrician*
   A doctor who specialises in the care of pregnant women and their babies.
e) *Gynaecologist*
   A doctor who specialises in the care of women during their reproductive years. A gynaecologist will attend the birth if the mother has been receiving treatment concerned with her reproductive system prior to, and during, pregnancy.
f) *Paediatrician*
   A doctor who specialises in the treatment of children's diseases. Most paediatricians work in hospital; some in the community.

THE ROLE OF THE FATHER DURING PREGNANCY AND BIRTH

In the latter part of the twentieth century it has become increasingly evident that the separate roles of father and mother are less distinct. It is now largely accepted practice that fathers take an active part in all aspects of the care and development of their children. Fathers who do this find parenting a much more rewarding experience and family relationships are closer as a result.

During pregnancy

a) Prepare for the experience of becoming a parent by reading, talking to relatives and friends, and attending antenatal classes.
b) Go with the mother to see the doctor and midwife who will be attending the birth so there is a firm relationship.
c) Visit the hospital, particularly the maternity unit, so that there is the best possible co-operation.
d) In some hospitals it is not usual for the father to attend the birth. If this is desired, ask permission.
e) Help with breathing and relaxation exercises.
f) Help the mother feel attractive and desirable, give reassurance, anticipate wishes, be aware of mood changes, cope with the lack of sexual response.
g) Act as a barrier to old wives' tales, with the help of relatives.
h) Go shopping together to choose baby equipment and toys, and clothes for the mother and baby.
i) Prepare the baby's room or area.
j) Towards the end of the pregnancy check the car over each morning for a full petrol tank, pressure in tyres; have pillows and blankets in car; find and practise the shortest route to hospital; know where the admission desk is. If no car – list telephone numbers of hospital, friends or reliable taxi companies.
k) Prepare room if home confinement.
l) Try to ensure that both sets of grandparents are involved.

Birth

If allowed to be present during labour and birth, the father can comfort the mother and give support and encouragement.

Immediately after the birth

The father should try to ensure that the mother holds the baby close as soon as possible, holds the baby himself and makes a request to be left with mother and baby to adjust to parenthood.

At home
The father should:
a) learn to care for the baby together with the mother, i.e. holding, comforting, feeding, dressing, playing, communicating, taking out;
b) make mother feel attractive and wanted; not pay too much attention to the baby at the expense of the mother; see that the mother gets plenty of rest; give support and be aware of possible postnatal depression;
c) go out with the mother, even for a short time, leaving the baby with some responsible adult;
d) not be jealous of time the mother spends with the baby;
e) not complain about the state of the house, help with the housework and encourage the return to normal routine;
f) give support to the mother if she gets up in the night to feed, change and comfort the baby;
g) recognise that caring for a baby is physically and mentally demanding for both parents. Exercise tolerance and understanding.

FAMILY PLANNING

It is medically advisable for the health of the mother and the children not to have pregnancies too close together. Family planning advice is free under the National Health Service for anyone over the age of 16, married or unmarried. It is far better to get individual and professional advice than to rely on experiences of friends. All communication with various agencies should be confidential.

Current contraceptive methods

a) *needing medical advice* – pill/mini pill, interuterine device, diaphragm, injection, sterilisation.
b) *not needing medical advice* (but not considered as reliable as the above) – sheath, spermicide, withdrawal, rhythm method.

Latest developments

Some contraceptives are only in the research stage, others are being test marketed in strict, clinically controlled experiments:

Men – a pill for men; spermicide-coated sheath.

Women – nasal contraceptive; silicone vaginal ring; new-type pill; 'vacation' pill; post intercourse drug; sponge barrier method; litmus test for ovulation.

Men and Women – reversible sterilisation for both.

ABORTION

Was legalised under 1967 Abortion Act. It is dangerous and irresponsible unless carried out under strict medical supervision. It is against some religious codes of practice. There are legal conditions under which an abortion can take place:

a) Two doctors must certify, except in case of emergency.
b) When pregnancy is thought to be a damage to the mother's health mentally and/or physically, or a risk to her life.
c) When tests indicate malformation of the foetus.
d) Should be done before the twelfth week, or if not possible, no later than the twenty-fourth week. (**N.B.** development of foetus p. 9–10.)

GROWTH AND DEVELOPMENT OF THE BABY AND PRE-SCHOOL CHILD

To grow physically means to increase in size. To develop means to progress through a series of changes, each of which is preparatory for the next. Baby and child growth and development should be considered a continuous process. The *pattern* of growth and development is the same for all normal babies and children. It is the *rate* which varies as this is influenced by heredity, environment and experiences.

It is widely accepted that:

1. The first 5 years of a child's life are crucial and can influence life in the future.
2. Growth and development are influenced by parental care and home conditions.
3. To develop and learn effectively, a child's needs must be met.

a) food;	e) exercise;	i) guidance;
b) warmth;	f) talk;	j) independence;
c) cleanliness;	g) play;	k) protection from danger;
d) rest;	h) love;	l) stimulation.

Baby and Child Development

Age Range	Physical	Mental/Intellectual	Social	Emotional	Language
Birth to 2 months	Rapid growth rate from birth; no head control; sensitive to bright lights; sucking reflex; limb waving.	Learns will be picked up and fed.	Begins to watch faces; smiles.	Satisfaction; excitement.	Crying, cooing.
2–4 months	Gradually learns head control; follows movement with eyes; kicks; holds small objects.	Recognises familiar voices.	Begins to react to familiar people.	Satisfaction; excitement; delight; distress.	Makes first sounds -m-, -g-, -n-.
4–6 months	Holds head up; tries to roll over; hears more accutely and responds to sounds; sits with support.	Further sounds recognised; basic response to language.	Laughs; specific attachments develop.	Excitement; delight; distress; anger; fear; disgust.	Chuckles; makes first -d- sound.
7–9 months	Tries to sit unaided; reaches out and grasps with whole hand; teeth develop; bites and chews.	Responds to language.	Begins to respond to less familiar adults.	Excitement; delight; distress; anger; fear;	Begins to develop vocabulary –
9–12 months	Tries to crawl; tries to stand; can pass objects from one hand to other hand.	Further development in response to language.		disgust; affection; elation.	4–6 words.
12–15 months	Tries to walk; can point to objects; uses both hands freely.	Looks at simple pictures with interest; identifies simple objects.	A gradual widening of social contacts, but needs familiar adults to be close; can be possessive of people and objects.	More evidence of the above emotions.	Vocabulary expands noticeably.
15–20 months	Walks; learns to run; feeds self with spoon; scribbles.	Further developments in observation of pictures; identifies objects; identification of people develops.	Begins to play side by side with other children.		Attempts at singing; language more recognisable; uses verbs; vocabulary about 10 words.

Age Range	Physical	Mental/Intellectual	Social	Emotional	Language
20 months – 2 years	Learns to climb stairs; balance improves; builds tower of 6 bricks; uses fingers to turn pages in books; runs; growth rate slows down.	Imitates people; looks at pictures and associated words; follows simple sequence of events in a story.		Intensification of above emotions.	Speech more fluent; gradually improves use of verbs; nouns and verbs used together; vocabulary about 50 words; obeys commands.
2–3 years	Builds tower with 9 bricks; walks upstairs with one foot on each step alternately; pedals and steers tricycle; walks on tip toes; kicks ball; catches ball with 2 arms; sits with ankles crossed; holds pencil correctly; usually dry at night.	Begins to follow stories with simple plot; begins to practise quantity.	Begins to accept spending night with familiar adults; can rebuff strangers; can be shy; still plays at side of other children.	plus joy and jealousy.	Develops confidence in the use of language; converses with self; vocabulary approximately 800 words; increased use of verbs.
3–4 years	Washes and dries hands, brushes teeth, can dress self except for difficult fastenings, walks up and down stairs, sits with knees crossed, throws and catches ball, runs on tiptoe, can stand on one leg for 5 seconds, builds bridge with bricks.	Follows stories about places in wider environment; begins to respond to simple humour; matches and names 4 colours.	Begins to play with other children; starts to develop give and take relationships with brothers and sisters; often develops an imaginary friend.	Additional emotions – hope; envy; anxiety;	Questions; progresses in sentence length; can state name and address; tell stories; uses pronouns; uses some prepositions.
4–5 years	Walks in straight line; can stand on one leg for 10 seconds; can thread needle and sew; draws house; copies a square; dresses and undresses; feeds self with knife and fork.	Imaginary play develops; obeys simple rules; begins to differentiate between fact and fantasy; names more than 4 colours; further application of vocabulary.	Plays with other children longer; shows off.	shame; disappointment.	Uses present and past tense; vocabulary approximately 1,500–2,000 words; uses longer sentences; word order more correct; wider use of adjectives; increased use of questions; clear and distinct speech.

The chart on pages 16 and 17 is a guide as to what an average child should be able to do at various ages. Parents should have some knowledge of the developmental stages so that they can provide the necessary conditions to aid development. The Clinic and Health Visitor will carry out assessment tests periodically to check that the child is progressing. If development is hindered in some way, further tests can be done to try and find the cause, so that treatment can be started.

THE ROLE OF PARENTS IN THE DEVELOPMENT OF THE PRE-SCHOOL CHILD

Parents should have some knowledge of developmental stages so that they can provide the necessary conditions to aid the development of the pre-school child. If the child has younger brothers or sisters, or close contact with other children, particularly older children, then development is usually helped because there is another child to imitate. For an only child, some contact with other children should be arranged and parents have more responsibility if this cannot be done.

INTELLECTUAL DEVELOPMENT

At this stage it is mainly the development of communication.

Talking and telling stories (from birth); having stories or poetry read.
Reading books – at first this will be play. Word recognition.
Writing. Holding writing tools and 'pretend' writing can help with later writing.
Counting by parents; child with parents; child alone.

Books, pictures, posters, friezes in the home help development if used wisely.

N.B. Parents can help intellectual development but care must be taken not to put undue pressure on children.

PHYSICAL DEVELOPMENT

At this stage it is mainly the development of manipulative skills and co-ordination of movement.

Grasping objects leading to development of placing, turning, grasping and holding toys, cutlery and cups.

Opening and closing movements, e.g. putting on clothes, fastening buttons and zips.

Body and limb movements and co-ordination, e.g. waving limbs, turning over, sitting up, crawling, standing, walking, running.

Touch, touching and stroking people and surfaces; interest in, and recognition of surfaces.

Parents can help physical development by providing opportunities – playing with children; providing simple toys which involve placing, turning, threading, etc.

SOCIAL DEVELOPMENT

At this stage it is a response to people and preparation for living.

Recognition – smiling, accepting body contacts, stretching out arms, waving goodbye, hugging, kissing, etc.

Playing with adults and other children.

Toilet training – recognition of discomfort by child, informing parent, asking for potty, going to lavatory.

Washing – water play, wiping hands on flannel, washing hands and face, cleaning teeth.

Meal times – feeding by parent, eating with fingers, spoon/pusher, cutlery, 'drinking cup' to normal cup.

Social contact – greetings, thank-you's, entertaining other children and adults.

Discipline – acceptable social behaviour needs to be fostered. Disciplining a young child should involve example, encouragement and warning. Punishment should be according to the age of the child and his or her ability to understand the reason for the punishment.

Independence – baby toilet seats, child's feeding utensils, clothes which are easy to put on and remove, social contacts with children and adults.

Attendance at nursery school or play group is usually an advantage for pre-school children both for social contacts and to help development. Children who have had opportunities to develop skills usually find school life easier.

MODULE TWO　REFERENCES

Magazines

Parents.
Mother & Baby.
Nursery World – leaflet service.
Family Circle.
Living.
Good Housekeeping – leaflet service.
N.A.M.C.W. publications.
F.P.A. publications.

Books

Life Before Birth S. Parker (C.U.P.)
Birth without Violence F. Leboyer (Fontana)
Pregnancy month by month (Consumers' Association)
The Experience of Childbirth S. Kitzinger (Pelican)
The Good Birth Guide S. Kitzinger (Fontana)
The Complete book of Babycare Ed. B. Nash (Octopus)
Child Care & Health for nursery nurses J. Brain and M. D. Martin (Hulton)

FOLLOW-UP ACTIVITIES

1. Invite a health visitor to discuss child growth and development.
2. List the advantages and disadvantages of a home versus hospital birth.
3. Which kinds of antenatal classes are available in your area and what is included in the classes?
4. Invite a group of mothers and babies to discuss growth and development.
5. Find out some of the differences/similarities between being a parent now and 50 years ago.
6. Select some books which are suitable for reading with the pre-school child.
7. Prepare a story to tell, or read a story from a book, to a young child.
8. Help a child to practise counting.

BABY AND CHILD CARE

Parenting is the knowledge, skills and attitudes which are developed by parents during the upbringing of their children. It involves being adaptable and flexible so that the needs of the individual child are met. For some parenting is easy; for others it is difficult; for all it is demanding. Providing for the physical needs of a new baby can be expensive. Unless there is planning, much time, energy and money can be wasted.

GENERAL GUIDELINES

a) Work out the amount of money available for equipment, etc.
b) Begin shopping in mid-pregnancy and try to complete by the eighth month.
c) Consider maintenance – washability, durability, design, comfort and safety.
d) Ask friends who have recently had babies which items were good value, useful, or useless.

NURSERY

A new baby needs a room, or an area of a room, and clothing and equipment for feeding, sleeping, bathing and exercise.
There should be:
a) Adequate storage space for clothing and equipment.
b) A maintained temperature of 21°C for the first two weeks of life, then 18°C. A separate heating appliance should conform to safety standards.
c) Adequate, draught-free ventilation and a moist atmosphere.
d) Safety locks on windows.

e) Flame-resistant or flameproof curtains or blind.
   N.B. Danger of plastic foams. (*Refer Book 2 – The Home*)
f) Hardwearing, comfortable, easy to clean floor covering.
g) Lighting which does not dazzle.
h) Stimulating, colourful, easy to clean wall and ceiling decor.

CLOTHING (*Refer Module 10*)

Weight of the baby is a better guide than size. First-size garments will fit a baby weighing up to 5·5 kg, second size up to 8 kg.
a) Have a minimum number of first-size garments.
b) Have at least one garment to wash, one to wear and one to air, except for nappies and waterproof pants.
c) Choose styles which give freedom of movement, have room for growth, are easy to put on and remove, have well-fitting cuffs, are not lacy to trap fingers and toes, have no 'fiddly' fastenings, are well made.
d) Choose fabrics which are machine washable, need little or no ironing, are shrink-resistant, dry quickly, are comfortable and suit the weather, are flame/fireproof.

Nappies

Choice is influenced by style of living, income and laundry facilities. They may be terry towelling squares, muslin squares, shaped towelling, disposable, combined disposable nappy and waterproof pants.
Waterproof pants may be pop on; tie on; pull on.

Suggested requirements for a new baby

24 terry squares
12 muslin squares (optional)
 3 pairs waterproof pants
 1 packet disposable nappies

1 packet safelock safety pins
1 packet nappy liner tissues
6 washable one-way liners

A typical layette will include

nappies and waterproof pants

vests

matinee coats

nightgowns

stretch towelling suits

pram sets

head wear (bonnets or helmets)

bootees

mittens

bibs

EQUIPMENT

a) *Feeding*

Bottle

6 bottles

6 teats (with different sized holes)

1 bottle brush

large container for sterilising *or* 1 steriliser unit

1 packet sterilising tablets

1 pot of salt to clean teats

1 spatula to level off scoops of feed

Breast

3 nursing bras

1 packet disposable breast pads

1 tube lanolin-based cream

In addition, 2 bottles and 2 teats to be used for water, expressed breast milk, and fruit juice.

b) *Sleeping*

Until baby weighs 9 kg, a large drawer (padded inside) or crib or carry cot is adequate. There are no set sleeping patterns. If there appears to be excessive or insufficient sleep, seek advice.

From about 4–5 months needs are:

cot and mattress to required safety standards

2 rubber under sheets

4 sheets (flannelette/knitted cotton/terry towelling)

2 cellular blankets *or*

2 duvets instead of top sheets

Fabrics should be machine washable and flame/fireproof.

c) *Bathing*
1 large washing up bowl *or*
1 baby bath.
2 buckets for wet and soiled nappies
1 bottle sterilising solution
1 PVC apron

2 soft terry towels
2 large plastic water jugs (hot and cold)
toiletries: all-in-one baby bath solution, nappy area cream, cotton wool

d) *Exercise*
Cost and style of living will influence choice.

1 pram conforming to safety standards: i.e. stability, locking device on brakes, safety harness and attachment, springing, depth, length, and convenient height for *both* parents (**N.B.** cat net attachment)
1 sun canopy if summer baby
pram blanket/duvet
1 rubber sheet
2 under sheets
1 carry cot and harness for back seat of car
1 playpen (**N.B.** safety standards)

When baby can sit up unsupported:
1 push chair (conforming to safety standards) with waterproof covering
1 baby sling or carrier
1 baby walker (**N.B.** safety standards)
1 safety seat for back of car

CARING GUIDELINES

It takes time to establish some kind of routine. During late pregnancy it is advisable to discuss and list which jobs are essential, important, or can be safely left until more time is available. What is vital is that parents should communicate with their baby during waking hours. Communicating means smiling, touching, cuddling, stroking, as well as talking and singing.

Feeding

The decision to breast or bottle feed should be taken in the last 3 months of pregnancy because the breasts need special care and preparation for breast feeding. Advice given in hospitals about breast feeding will vary and is often conflicting. There is no doubt that breast milk is usually better and the source of supply is readily available. But not every mother wants to breast feed and not every mother can. If the baby is bottle fed, take advice from the health visitor about the choice of the food and follow instructions about preparation rigidly.

Feeding time for a young baby offers an opportunity for body contact with the parent, providing satisfaction, reassurance, warmth and love.

WEANING

Weaning means getting the child used to taking other foods besides milk. It is best not to start weaning from breast or bottle until the baby is about 6 months old; never before 3 months old. Commercially prepared weaning foods are best, simplest and safest. Follow advice from the health visitor.

Feeding during weaning should also be a pleasurable time for the baby and parents.

CRYING

Babies cry for various reasons:

soiled nappy | thirst
wet nappy | hunger
boredom | heat
loneliness | cold
exhaustion | illness

Check for:
a) thirst – give freshly boiled, cooled water;
b) wet or soiled nappy;
c) boredom or loneliness;
d) *then* for hunger.
NB Teething should be a normal proceess. If there appears to be a lot of discomfort, seek advice.

NAPPY CHANGING

Never delay changing a soiled or wet nappy; it is uncomfortable and distressing for the baby and can cause chafing or skin rashes. There is no correct way to put on a terry napkin – use a safe method which provides most absorbency and is comfortable. Follow the instructions of the health visitor.

Guidelines

a) wash hands;
b) collect equipment: clean nappy, clean liner, cotton wool, oil/lotion/cream, safety pins;
c) put baby on back on safe flat surface, remove waterproof pants, unfasten nappy;
d) if bottom is soiled, gently wipe away mess (from front to back) with tissue or corner of nappy;
e) wipe bottom clean (front to back) with cotton wool and lotion or water;
f) smooth lotion/cream on bottom gently;
g) allow baby to kick for a few minutes to let air get to skin;
h) lift baby on to clean nappy and liner, secure in place;
i) put on waterproof pants and put baby in safe place;
j) dispose of soiled or wet nappy (see below);
k) wash your hands.

Nappy laundering

a) every morning make up fresh sanitising solution in 2 buckets; wash hands;
b) rinse *wet* nappies in cold running water; soak for at least 2 hours in one bucket;
c) hold *soiled* nappies under flushing water of lavatory; soak for at least 2 hours in another bucket;
d) rinse nappies from 'wet bucket'; dry (never on radiator – makes them stiff);
e) wash nappies from 'soiled bucket' according to Label 1. wash code (*Refer Book 2 – The Home*) put to dry (outdoor drying is preferable);
f) do not use strong disinfectants.

It is obvious that disposable nappies save time and effort, but many parents prefer the traditional nappies which are also cheaper to use.

BATHING

Some parents prefer to bath the baby in the morning, others at night; either is correct, but baby needs a bath every day, unless this is against medical advice.

a) Collect equipment: bath, water (hot and cold), cotton wool, clean clothes, nappy changing equipment, baby bath lotion/soap, brush, comb, nail scissors, small basin of cool boiled water, towel, PVC apron.

b) Ensure room is warm and draught-free.

c) Have bottle near if bottle-fed.

d) Put on apron and wash hands.

e) Put cold water in bath, add hot water until temperature is warm (38°C) – the traditional method for testing is by the parent's elbow because it is sensitive to temperature. A special card thermometer is now available.

f) Undress baby except for nappy, and wrap in towel with arms inside and put on flat surface.

g) Use a small swab of clean cotton wool, dampened with cool boiled water from basin, and gently wipe one eye from nose outwards; take clean dry swab and wipe same eye again. Repeat procedure with other eye using *fresh* swabs.

h) Wash face with damp swab, dry gently with corner of towel; *do not poke up nose or in ears*; wipe gently with tightly wrung-out swab and dry gently.

i) Hold baby under one arm supporting head and shoulders, hold over bath; use free hand to scoop water over hair and wash gently; rinse well and pat dry.

j) Put baby on flat surface, remove towel and nappy; put used nappy in bucket; clean bottom gently.

k) Lift baby into bath with both hands and hold securely in a half-sitting position; scoop water over body and allow baby to kick and splash for a few minutes; if using soap, parent should soap hands and massage gently all over baby's body *before* putting into bath. If unsure, have the help of a responsible person at this stage – also at any other stage if necessary.

l) Lift out on to towel and wrap loosely.

m) Pat dry; pay attention to folds of skin.

n) Cream bottom; put on clean nappy.

o) Put on required clothing and feed.

p) When baby is settled, dispose of used swabs, bath water, soiled or wet nappy, used clothing (hygienically and tidily).

N.B. Bathing can be a dangerous procedure; follow the advice and instructions of the health visitor carefully.

IMMUNISATION

A precaution against certain diseases. The service is easily obtained through the Health Service, usually from the clinic, and it is free of charge.

Guidelines

1st year				2nd year		3rd year	4th year	5th year
3 mths	6 mths	9 mths	12 mths	15 mths	18 mths			
D. T. (P.) polio	D. T. (P.)	polio	D. T. (P.) polio	measles german measles mumps T.B. test	D. T. polio			boosters for: D. T. polio

D – diptheria
T – tetanus   } called the
P – pertusis – whooping cough   } 'Triple vaccine'

If travelling abroad the child may also need protection against: smallpox, typhoid, yellow fever, cholera.

Sometimes there can be side effects. It is unusual for them to be serious. The protection far outweighs the risk of side effects.

CARE OF BOTH PARENTS

This aspect of child care is often overlooked. Bringing up and caring for babies and children is demanding and if both parents are not healthy then they cannot hope to cope successfully.

Guidelines

Correct diet; adequate rest; pride in appearance; get out of the house daily for exercise and stimulation; chat to other parents out with their babies and children – they may be lonely.

PLAY AND TOYS

Play is the child's work and toys are the tools. It is through play that the child's whole development may be encouraged. The child can make use of all the senses (hearing, sight, touch, smell and taste) during play activities.

This is a general pattern; some children vary in the activities related to the age range and many activities are on-going through the age range.

Age Range	Play Materials and Toys
Birth–3 months	Self, parents, rattles, squeaky toys, cuddly toys.
3–6 months	Rattles, teething rings, balls, floating toys in bath.
6–9 months	Push-along toys. Stacking toys.
9–12 months	Push–pull toys. Books with everyday objects. Fitting blocks and shapes together.
12–18 months	Books with pictures including objects outside the home. Sand pit and paddling pool – under supervision.
18 months– 2 years	Stories with simple events (shopping, zoo, birthday party). Dressing up. Books with a few words per page.
2–3 years	Clay, dough, plasticene, jugs, cups, beakers, musical instruments, painting, large crayons.
3–4 years	Stories with simple plot. Tricycles, pedal cars, dolls, animals, prams, simple puzzles.
4–5 years	Dolls houses, cars, garages, trains, farms, zoos, tea sets. Simulated household utensils and household tasks. More complex stories.

The baby's first toy is his own body; he will gradually explore it, using all his senses. The second toy is his parents; he will explore their faces and bodies in the same way. Unless parents are aware of this fact, they can deprive their child and themselves of a valuable experience.

There are four stages of play through which every child passes:
a) solitary – plays alone;
b) parallel – plays by the side of other children;
c) simple co-operative – begins to join in play activities of other children;
d) complex co-operative – joins fully in play activities of other children.

All toys sold in United Kingdom are subject to strict safety regulations but a check should be made. A good toy is:

fun	safe
stimulating and rewarding	durable
well-designed and constructed	good value for money
brightly coloured	suitable for age and ability of child
interestingly textured	hygienic.

From an early age the child should be encouraged to put toys away tidily at the end of playtime.

SAFETY IN THE HOME

Every year many children die or are seriously injured as a result of accidents in the home. Those children at greatest risk are under four years old because they are naturally curious, they copy adults, and they do not understand the meaning of danger.

Children need to be protected by making the home environment secure and free from hazards. Adults must reinforce warnings by setting a good example. There must be positive, continuous teaching of safety to develop safe habits.

COMMUNITY PROVISION FOR UNDER FIVES

The different forms of child care in the community are the responsibility of the local authority. Provision varies greatly from authority to authority. *Advantages* include opportunities to mix with other children and adults, the development of independence and self-confidence, enjoyment of a wider range of play activities. (Refer to chart on page 31.)

Type	Age	Premises	Hours	Cost	Local Authority Department Responsible	Staff
Nursery school	3 & 4 years.	Nursery school.	Monday–Friday; 2 daily sessions; school terms; attend am or pm.	Free.	Education.	Nursery nurse; nursery teacher; (1 adult to 10/12 children).
Nursery class	4 years.	Nursery or infant school.	As nursery school.	Free.	Education.	Teacher – not always specially trained.
Day nursery	Few weeks–school age.	Day nursery.	Daily 07.30–17.30; not public holidays.	Varies with need and income of parents.	Social Services.	Matron; nurse; nursery nurse; teacher; aide.
Playgroup	3 & 4 years.	Custom built; church hall; village hall; private house.	Varies: a) daily; b) mornings; c) afternoons; d) once a week; e) twice weekly.	Varies; sometimes social services pay for children in need.	Must be registered with Social Services.	Untrained leader; trained leader; parents on rota; (1 adult to 8 children).
Child minder	Few weeks–school age.	Private home.	By arrangement with parents.	Negotiated according to provision.	By law must be registered with Social Services.	Child minder must have a) medical and chest X-ray b) *never* had a child removed from care by Local Authority c) *never* been convicted of an offence against a child.

MODULE THREE REFERENCES

Magazines
(Refer Module 2)

Books
The Newborn Baby (Consumers' Association)
The Experience of Breastfeeding S. Kitzinger (Pelican)
Breast is Best P. & A. Stanway (Pan)
Reader's Digest Mothercare Book
Who wants to cook? M. Philip (Heinemann)
Cooking for a baby S. Hull (Mother & Baby)
Baby and Child Penelope Leach (Michael Joseph)

Booklets
'*What every Mum and Dad should know about British Standards*' (British Standards Institution: Education Section)

FOLLOW-UP ACTIVITIES

1. Make a toy which is planned for safety. Explain why it should be safe.
2. Investigate the safety points to look for in a playpen; pram; cot; push-chair.
3. Make up a bottle for a baby weighing 12 lb/5.4 kg.
4. Carry out a costing exercise on basic equipment for a new baby.
5. Find out the differences and similarities in child care practices 100 years ago and today.
6. Visit a library or museum to find out what children's clothing and equipment was like in past centuries.
7. Carry out an investigation on a child's toy; report your findings.
8. Invite the health visitor to discuss and demonstrate procedures in the care of a baby.
9. Visit a day nursery/playgroup and note the activities of the children. Talk to a nurse or playgroup leader; report on your findings.
10. Plan the meals for a toddler for one week.
11. Invite a small group of young children and their parents to school. Discuss their care routines. Serve refreshments.

CHILDHOOD TO ADULTHOOD

CHILDHOOD TO THE ONSET OF PUBERTY

The age group is approximately 6–11 years (the primary school age group). Children of the same age group show great differences in development.

PHYSICAL DEVELOPMENT

There will be much variation in size and weight. Girls usually grow at a faster rate than boys during this period. There is great activity. Group games are popular. Muscle co-ordination develops and movements become more skilled. Puberty may commence. Much health care is needed and sound nutrition.

INTELLECTUAL DEVELOPMENT

Most important stage in overall intellectual development. The basic skills need to be acquired – reading; writing; numbers; communication/use of language. Much memorising is required and reasoning ability should develop. Creative skills may be revealed, e.g. music. This is a period of curiosity and discovery. The effects of television viewing need to be considered.

EMOTIONAL DEVELOPMENT

Most children are friendly and cheerful with a favourable attitude towards school. There is a gradual move away from too much dependence upon parents, towards friends outside the home, and towards independence.

SOCIAL DEVELOPMENT

There will have been different social experiences from babyhood, e.g. in mixing with other children in the family or at play group, etc. Some children will have developed independence, e.g. dressing; toilet training. Communication skills will vary. The move from the shelter of the home to contacts outside – school and the neighbourhood – is very difficult for some children. The solitary play of babyhood changes to group play although there may be a lot of reading. Again, the effects of television viewing need to be considered.

The period of childhood should include

a) Sound nutrition and attention to health.
b) The development of the habits of safety, hygiene, tidiness and helping at home (boys as well as girls).
c) Opportunities to develop independence.
d) Leisure activities with children of the same age group.
e) Full advantage of educational opportunities.
f) Love and guidance from the home.
g) Protection by society.

PUBERTY TO ADOLESCENCE

This is the period of life where there is most physical and emotional change and the interaction of one upon another. There is a need for knowledge and understanding by the person involved, the family, friends, school and society.

Puberty
The word comes from the Latin 'pubertas' – the age of manhood, when sexual functions mature.

Adolescence
This is usually defined as the period of transition between childhood and adulthood. It includes the period of puberty and lasts until adulthood and is considered to cover the period of 12 years to 20 years. As in the earlier stage of childhood, there are variations in the timing of developments.

PHYSICAL DEVELOPMENT

General development

Period of most change. There are variations in growth and in body size and shape. Girls may be taller at the beginning of this period because the growth spurt was earlier, but boys develop rapidly usually at about 13 years. Size and build are affected by heredity (inherited genes). Malnutrition, illness and functional diseases, and handicap can inhibit growth. The skin may be affected by over production from the sebaceous glands, resulting in enlarged pores, blackheads, acne and greasy hair.

Sexual development

The process of development takes from 2 to 5 years. Some adolescents may have completed the development at the age when another is at the first stage. This does not affect final development. Hormone activity of sex glands (gonads) influences physical growth and sexual development. Sexual development usually follows a pattern.

BOYS
a) Testes and scrotum increase in size.
b) Pubic hair begins to appear.
c) Penis increases in size. Production of seminal fluid begins.
d) The voice begins to deepen as the larynx grows and the vocal cords lengthen. It may take 2 years for complete deepening to occur.
e) Seminal fluid containing sperms is produced in more quantity. Nocturnal emission may occur.
f) Axillary (underarm) hair develops and hair grows on the face.
g) Pubic hair becomes pigmented.

GIRLS
a) Beginning of breast development – 'bud' development.
b) Rounding of hips.
c) Pubic hair begins to appear.
d) Increase in the size of genital organs.
e) Development of pigmented pubic hair.
f) Development of axillary hair.
g) Further development of breasts.
h) Menarche – onset of menstruation.
i) Further maturation of breasts and growth of axillary hair.

Menstruation

Onset of menstruation is almost always after the peak growth in height. It usually starts about the age of 12 or 13 years but sometimes is as early as 9 or 10 years or as late as 15 or 16 years. The late start may be the result of late development, illness or malnutrition.

The monthly cycle of menstruation is controlled by hormones in the pituitary gland. An egg (ovum) is released from an ovary and passes along the fallopian tube to be available for fertilisation. There is the capability to conceive about a year after the menarche. When fertilisation does not occur, the egg and the lining of the uterus are passed out of the body through the vagina. The menstrual flow, which is composed of blood, mucin and cells, usually lasts 4 to 5 days but may be shorter or longer.

Menstrual protection may be by pads or tampons made from absorbent cellulose material. Pads are held inside briefs by ties or adhesive strips. Tampons are inserted into the vagina by means of an applicator and removed by the attached cord. It is vital that strict hygiene is observed before and after insertion as there could be a danger of infection. Sanitary protection should be changed as soon as necessary. At the beginning of the period, the flow is likely to be heavier and a change needed every 3 to 4 hours. More absorbent pads and tampons can be obtained.

Cleanliness is important during menstruation. A bath, shower or all-over wash should be taken each day. It is quite safe to wash hair. Used pads should be wrapped and burned or placed in a sanitary bin. Used tampons may be flushed away.

Exercise should be taken normally. Swimming is possible if tampons are worn but care should be taken if there is a heavy discharge. Do not swim if conditions are very cold.

Cramp and pain may occur during a period. This may be caused by lack of exercise, bad posture or malnutrition. Specialist help should be obtained for particular problems.

Depression or stress may occur but this should only be slight. If deeper depression occurs, specialist help should be obtained.

Menopause (change of life) is the end of menstruation and the end of the body's reproductive function. It usually occurs during the mid-forties or early fifties.

INTELLECTUAL DEVELOPMENT

The years between childhood and adulthood are important in intellectual development. The development of intellectual potential may depend upon the opportunities provided – in the home, in school and in the environment, and also on the willingness of the individual to take advantage and profit by the opportunities offered. In the past, some school subjects tended to be recommended for either boys or girls. To some extent this still occurs, i.e. some science subjects, especially physics, are considered more suited to boys because of the expectations of society in general and parents in particular. The need to obtain qualifications is a serious consideration in later adolescence.

EMOTIONAL DEVELOPMENT

This is a period of much emotional fluctuation, mainly because of the many physical changes, particularly those concerned with sexual development. There may be quick changes of mood from overexcitement to depression which need not be of concern provided that there is no deep and lasting depression and withdrawal. The desire to be independent is strong and yet the need for guidance and security is still present. This may result in defiant behaviour or exhibitionism, to try to prove that childhood is passed. Some adolescents are attracted to 'causes', religions or cults and in some cases deep involvement has caused problems. There may be difficulties in relationships at home or at school but with support from the family and friends most adolescents are able to cope with emotional changes.

SOCIAL DEVELOPMENT

As there is such a wide variation in the rate of development, some adolescents are suited to certain social activities perhaps nearer to those of an adult, while other adolescents of the same age group are drawn to more youthful social activities. At the beginning of the adolescent period, many boys still prefer to be in male groups but gradually groups become mixed and smaller groupings and pairings occur. There may be insecurity with the opposite sex because of lack of contact earlier in life or because there are few opportunities for social mixing.

Adolescents need to learn to 'fit in' with the customs and rules of the society in which they live or there could be problems. This can be particularly difficult when the family originated from a different culture and the children are living between two types of society with different customs.

The period of adolescence should include

a) Sound nutrition and attention to health.
b) Family support, love and guidance.
c) Leisure activities and friendship of people in the same age group.
d) Education for intellectual, physical and social development.
e) Protection and acceptance by society.
f) Co-operation by the adolescent with society, school and family.

YOUNG ADULTHOOD

This is the period between adolescence and full adulthood. The age range is approximately 20 to 25 years. There is a wide variety of occupations and social relationships – work or unemployment; left school at 16 years or in full-time education; unmarried; married; divorced. Individuals may be living in the parental home or in independent accommodation. Married couples may have a home of their own or live with parents and there may be one or more children of the marriage. By the end of this stage of development, people should have obtained physical maturity, but will have had varying opportunities for intellectual, social and emotional development.

THE ADULT

An adult is considered to be a mature person who usually has the ability, gained by experience, to face realities, handle success or failure, and to make decisions.

MODULE FOUR   REFERENCES

The Developing Child H. Bee (Harper & Row)

FOLLOW-UP ACTIVITIES

1. Talk to adolescents from different cultures about their social activities and family expectations.
2. Talk to parents and grandparents about their experiences as adolescents.
3. Visit a primary school or talk to children of primary school age about their interests and the games that they play. Identify changes since you were in that age group.
4. List the advantages and disadvantages of television viewing for the young child.

THE ELDERLY

In this module the term 'the elderly' refers to the group of people who are of pensionable age. In the United Kingdom this refers to men of 65 years and over and women of 60 years and over. They comprise about 20 per cent of the total population of the UK. The percentage is increasing because people are living longer and are healthier because of:
a) Improved living and working conditions.
b) Advances in medicine.
c) Developments in the Public Health Services.
d) Better health education.

AGEING PROCESS

The process of ageing is not yet fully understood. It is variable both in its effects on individuals, its onset and pace of development. It must be appreciated that two elderly people of the same age may differ greatly in physical and mental health.

Features of the ageing process

a) Failing sight.
b) Hearing difficulties – can be due to wax build-up.
c) Gums shrink and dentures do not fit correctly, causing difficulty in eating (or teeth loosen).
d) Memory weakens.
e) Learning ability impaired, therefore hard to adapt to a new environment.
f) Decline in muscle strength.

g) Sense of smell reduced.
h) Hair loses its colour. It may fall out.
i) Sleep patterns affected.
j) Bones become brittle and break more easily.
k) Skin loses its elasticity and wrinkles develop.
l) Reduction in mobility, caused by heart disease, high blood pressure, rheumatism, arthritis, sight or hearing failure.
m) Loss of ability to react quickly.
n) Intellectual capacity can be reduced.
o) Repair after injury takes longer than in a youthful person.
p) Respiratory organs lose their efficiency and take longer to return to normal after exercise.
q) Infectious disease protection mechanism impaired.
r) When ill can take a long time for symptoms to show – by then the disease is often at the chronic stage and more difficult to treat.

NEEDS OF THE ELDERLY

1. Sufficient income.
2. Suitable and secure accommodation.
3. A well-balanced diet.
4. A comprehensive range of medical and community services.
5. Regular social contacts.
6. Feeling of dignity.
7. Degree of independence with protection.
8. Advice on preparation for retirement.

INCOME

Men who are 65 years old and women who are 60 years old are entitled to receive a state retirement pension if they have:
a) retired from regular employment;
b) satisfied the state contribution conditions.
If a person continues in paid employment over 70 years of age for a man and over 65 years for a woman, then retirement pension is payable in addition to the income received from the employer.

A married woman will receive a retirement pension on her husband's contribution record at 60 years if:
a) she has retired from paid employment;

b) her husband is 65 years and retired from paid employment;
c) her husband's contribution record is satisfactory.

A woman may also qualify for a retirement pension on her own contribution record at 60 years. If she qualifies on her own *and* her husband's record then she will receive
a) the higher pension; or
b) a combination of the two up to a stated maximum amount.

Since April 1978, retirement pensions comprise two parts:
   1. basic pension.   2. earnings related pension.

The scheme is inflation-protected and men and women receive equal treatment. It provides a retirement income similar to occupational pensions provided by certain employers. Women can now have their pension rights protected when they are absent from paid employment for childbearing.

SUITABLE ACCOMMODATION

Accommodation provision for this age group varies throughout the country. Many elderly are owner occupiers; some rent rooms, flats or houses privately; others rent from local authorities; some live with relations or are in residential care. It has been found that over 25 per cent of all households of this age group lack one basic amenity, e.g. no hot water; no inside lavatory.

Since 1969 there have been mandatory design standards for dwellings for the elderly which are owned by local authorities and housing associations:
a) category I – self-contained, one or two person dwellings, with or without a resident warden and with communal facilities nearby.
b) category II – flatlets for the less active members of this age group. There is an alarm system to alert a resident warden, and communal areas which are centrally heated to a required standard.

In both categories the design standards cover:

windows	cookers	siting of electric sockets	floors
doors	baths	door handles	shelving
stairs	lavatories	window catches	insulation

Some local authorities provide a grouped flatlet system with accommodation for either single persons or couples. The flatlets are let unfurnished and have communal facilities comprising sitting rooms, laundry rooms and store rooms. A resident warden is in attendance and is immediately available through an intercom link or an emergency call system.

Living with the family

Most elderly people prefer to live near to their relations rather than live with them. However, some old people become incapable of performing the tasks of everyday living. One alternative to this problem is to take them into the family unit. The possible effects of the decision can be far reaching and disruptive and must be carefully discussed with all concerned before it is undertaken.

SOME FACTORS AFFECTING THE DECISION
a) relationship involved;
b) physical health of elderly person(s);
c) mental state of elderly person(s);
d) size of the dwelling and number of family members;
e) ground floor accommodation;
f) alterations to the dwelling (e.g. extra handrails on the stairs, in the bath or separate or additional lavatory);
g) change in household expenditure.

Residential care

In this country may be in:
a) National Health Service hospitals.
b) Homes for the Elderly (private, voluntary, local authority).
c) Private nursing homes.
d) Homes/hostels for the physically/mentally handicapped.
The provision can be short-term or long-term depending on the frailty and disability of the elderly person. When considering this type of accommodation the following should be taken into account:
1. Obtain the best available professional advice.
2. Ascertain the full range of services available.
3. View the accommodation before making a decision.
4. Find out how free a life the elderly person is able to lead.
5. Ascertain the qualifications of the staff.
6. Is there access to the shops and the community?
7. What are the facilities for making hot drinks, etc?
8. Can the bed times be chosen?
9. Is there free and private access to the telephone?
10. Are guests received/entertained in private?

11. Is there a choice of bedroom, diet, medical care?

12. What is the provision for elderly members of different ethnic groups? Can they follow their own cultural traditions, religious affiliations and dietary preferences?

13. What is the cost?

14. What entertainment is available?

15. Do the residents appear to be happy and contented?

A WELL-BALANCED DIET

The interest that this age group takes in food is related to income, mental activity, adjustment to old age, loneliness and level of mobility. If the person has the ability to budget, to select and prepare food, has a good adjustment to present life and is mobile, then the interest in eating is usually high and health is correspondingly good. The role of a well-balanced diet in preventive medicine is assuming increasing importance.

COMPREHENSIVE RANGE OF MEDICAL AND COMMUNITY SERVICES

Generally, the health and social services work closely with voluntary agencies to provide a full range of services in the community. Difficulties arise because many elderly people are unaware of what is available, where to go to get advice and how to take up the services provided. In areas where a large number of elderly people tend to retire, the services may be stretched beyond their capacity.

a) *Medical service personnel*

In each community there is a Primary Health Care team comprising general practitioners, district nurses, health visitors. Other medical services include: dentists, opticians, pharmacists, chiropodists, physiotherapists.

b) *Social Services personnel*

social workers, home helps, meals-on-wheels workers, mobility officers for the blind, advisers on technical aids, occupational therapists, day centre personnel (with voluntary aid).

c) *Voluntary agency services*

shopping, changing library books, cooking, gardening, household tasks, decorating, chopping firewood, social interaction.

There is liaison with medical and social service personnel. The local Citizens

Advice Bureau will be able to give information on the statutory and voluntary services available in the community.

REGULAR SOCIAL CONTACTS

Elderly people living alone tend to suffer from loneliness and boredom. A contributory factor to loneliness may be due to a lack of family support because:
a) they never married;
b) they were childless;
c) their children and grandchildren live some distance away;
d) the spouse is dead;
e) retirement was into a new environment;
f) they have an inability to make new friends.

Mobility can influence the number of available social contacts in the community. Social contact is sought through:
a) shopping – the more mobile go to the shops daily;
b) visiting relations who live nearby;
c) visiting friends who live nearby;
d) attending a day centre, Darby & Joan Club, over 60's club or recreational classes;
e) attending church;
f) hobbies;
g) holidays.

Those who are unable to leave the home and whose relatives live at a distance may rely very heavily on the voluntary and statutory service sectors of the community for their social contact. Unfortunately, their needs are not always met adequately. Television and radio are all too often the only ways of relieving the boredom and the loneliness of some old people.

FEELING OF DIGNITY

In countries where the kinship network is strong and supportive, the elderly are treated with respect and accorded high status in the family structure. They are deemed to have wisdom and experience in dealing with the problems of life. Their advice on family and community matters is sought often and freely given. Many become tribal elders. In many Western cultures this does not happen. The elderly as a social group tend to be treated as children or neglected and are seen as a burden to the family and to a society whose emphasis is on youth.

DEGREE OF INDEPENDENCE

Freedom to make decisions about daily living is important to all age groups in society but especially to the elderly. They do need support from various social agencies as well as from their families and friends but they do not want their lives organised without consultation.

ADVICE AND PREPARATION FOR RETIREMENT

Women tend to find retirement easier to adapt to than men. As the roles of men and women in marriage become increasingly shared this may not be a problem for the future generations of elderly people. The health of some people at the age of 65 years has so deteriorated that they are only suited to a very leisurely retirement. Others remain physically and mentally active and adapt successfully to the process of ageing.

It has been found that preparation for retirement needs to be started in the last decade of paid employment since retirement involves both changes in attitudes and changes in lifestyle.

Increasingly, employers, trade unions, local education authorities and voluntary bodies are setting up courses and counselling for the period of retirement. These services provide information on:
a) budgeting on a reduced income;
b) moving to a smaller residence which is easier to maintain;
c) diet management;
d) simple keep-fit programmes;
e) leisure activities;
f) bereavement counselling;
g) statutory and voluntary agencies to help with problems which may arise.

Unsuccessful adaptation to retirement and old age is caused by:
a) failure to keep up with the world outside the home;
b) loss of youthful vigour;
c) loss of stable emotional relationships – departure of children, death of spouse or other relatives and friends;
d) unsuitable accommodation;
e) mismanagement of reduced income;
f) loneliness;
g) loss of work status, interest and associates;

h) feeling of uselessness;
i) lack of hobbies/outside interests.

Elderly members of ethnic minority groups may face additional problems caused by different cultural traditions and language difficulties. There needs to be an appreciation of their difficulties by the Social Services.

Successful adaptation to retirement and old age is caused by:
a) satisfactory social relationships;
b) adequate plans for retirement years;
c) inner satisfaction with life;
d) functional capacity being maintained;
e) financial security;
f) suitable accommodation and the ability to manage;
g) personal interests.

NATIONAL VOLUNTARY SOCIETIES CONCERNED WITH THE ELDERLY

Age Concern
Elderly Invalids' Fund
Friends of the Elderly and Gentlefolks' Help
Help the Aged
Sisters of Our Lady of Grace and Compassion
Preretirement Association.

Growing old need not be a time of loneliness and boredom. Elderly people who are happy and well-adjusted have friends and close family relationships and interests. They are not dependent upon previous employment or youthful vigour.

CRIME AND THE ELDERLY

Crimes against the elderly are on the increase, particularly physical attacks either in the home or in the street. It is vital that the elderly are helped to appreciate the dangers and plan their way of life accordingly. They should *not*:

a) open the door to strangers;
b) keep large amounts of money or valuables in the house;
c) carry money and valuables around with them;
d) walk alone at night, or in certain areas during the day;
e) be afraid to seek advice from the police about home security arrangements.

The following handout has been issued by the Merseyside Police to help the public as well as the elderly appreciate the dangers.

CRIME
and the
ELDERLY

Merseyside Police are at present running a campaign which seeks to:-

* Make elderly people more crime prevention conscious.

* Encourage neighbourly concern to increase the elderly person's sense of security.

* Hopefully allay some exaggerated fears about crime.

* To advise elderly people just what they can do to reduce the risks of their becoming a victim of crime.

If you would like to discuss your own security, contact your local police station and ask for the CRIME PREVENTION OFFICER.

His advice is free - it may save you from becoming another victim of crime.

Issued by the Merseyside Police Crime Prevention Department. (1981)

MODULE FIVE   REFERENCES

The Old in the Community (Help the Aged Education Department)
1981 Guide to the Social Services (Family Welfare Association)
Voluntary Social Services Directory (Bedford Square Press)

FOLLOW-UP ACTIVITIES

1. Design a flat suitable for an elderly person.
2. Find out more about the design standards for purpose-built accommodation for the elderly.
3. Imagine you are a member of a local authority housing committee planning the siting of accommodation for elderly people. Write down the factors affecting the choice of the site.
4. Consider the factors affecting the family when an elderly relative comes to live in the family home.
5. Talk to elderly persons about their childhood. Compare with your own experiences.
6. Visit a Day Centre in your community and talk to the elderly people there. Write an account of your findings.
7. Find out about the 'adopt a grannie/grandad scheme'. Does one operate in your community?
8. Plan and cost the menus for a week for an elderly person living alone.
9. Invite a group of elderly people to school for coffee, lunch or afternoon tea.

HEALTH

HISTORY

The World Health Organisation has defined health as being 'A state of complete physical, mental and social well-being and not simply the absence of disease or infirmity'. Health should be considered by the individual, the family and the community – local, national and global. Ill health causes physical and mental suffering, and it is costly in finance, time and effort.

At the present time, local authorities and governments, at national and international level, are concerned about standards of health. In the past, there were few positive approaches to the maintenance of health. Concern focussed on coping with diseases and epidemics such as plague, cholera, typhus, smallpox, tuberculosis and poliomyelitis. In 1348, the Black Death spread to Britain from Europe and is thought to have killed almost half the population. There were more outbreaks and then, in 1665, the Great Plague of London. The spread of the plague was stopped by the Great Fire of London in 1666 which destroyed unsanitary conditions.

Diseases causing illness and death continued through the centuries. Cholera was particularly dreaded and there were four serious outbreaks in Britain between 1830 and 1870, causing over 5,300 deaths in 1849. In the nineteenth century, other diseases such as typhus and smallpox caused a number of deaths, and tuberculosis, poliomyelitis, diphtheria, scarlet fever, influenza and dysentery were common in limited outbreaks or in epidemics. Prevention was mainly centred upon the isolation and avoidance of those suffering from disease – lepers were an early example. The need to identify the causes and transmission of diseases was only realised slowly.

The appalling standards of housing and sanitation was not generally thought to have any connection with disease. Sewage from London houses drained into the River Thames which, without purification, was the main water supply. The scarcity of water added to the filth and squalor. A number of streets in the poorer areas shared a single tap which was sometimes at a great distance. Atmospheric pollution by smoke and discharge from factories was a contributory factor in respiratory diseases. The effects of the increased concentration of pollution which occurs in fog or 'smog' (fog plus smoke) can be fatal. As late as 1952, over 4,000 deaths in London were attributed to a 'killer smog'.

Up to the end of the nineteenth century, medical knowledge was limited and medical care was often of a poor standard. Although there were some free dispensaries in cities, many poor people could not afford to take time off work or to meet the cost of travel. Thousands of people died because of diseases caused by unsanitary conditions, from malnutrition or under-nutrition, and from lack of medical attention. It is reported that in 1842 over half the children in British cities died before they reached the age of 5 years.

A number of people worked to try to reduce the high level of disease, e.g. Edward Jenner introduced vaccination against smallpox; Louis Pasteur discovered the relationship of bacteria to infection; Lord Lister introduced the use of antiseptics.

COMMUNITY ACTION

Public Health was not considered to be the concern of State or local authority and there were no effective sanitary provisions or housing legislation until late into the nineteenth century. The following are examples:

1848 Public Health Act	Districts 'encouraged' to take measures against unsanitary conditions. Sanctions after 1853.
1858 Medical Act	General Council of Medical Education and Registration established.
1869 Royal Sanitary Commission	Statement of a National Sanitary Minimum including: Supply of wholesome and sufficient water for drinking and washing. Provision of sewerage and the utilisation of sewage.

	Regulation of streets, highways and new building.
	The healthiness of dwellings.
	The removal of nuisances and refuse.
	The inspection of food.
	The suppression of causes of disease.
1875 Public Health Act	Recommendations of the Commission 1869 to be implemented. Local Authorities empowered to provide hospitals.
1897	First Health Visitor appointed in Liverpool.
1904 Report of the Committee on Physical Deterioration	Major health defects named: poor physical development; bad dentition; defective vision; heart disease.
1906 Education (Provision of Meals) Act	Local Authorities encouraged to provide meals for needy children.
1907 Education (Administrative Provisions) Act	Local Authorities to have elementary school children medically examined.
1911 National Health Insurance Act	Part I. Health Workers earning less than £3 a week to receive free medical attention and medicine and sick pay 7/– (35p) a week. Compulsory contributions by workers and employers. Part II. Unemployment Unemployment pay 7/– (35p) a week for 15 weeks. Contributions from workers and employers. Only covered a few industries in the beginning. (In both Part I and Part II payments the State makes up the contributions to full cost.)
1918 Maternal and Child Welfare Act	Local Authorities empowered to safeguard the health of expectant mothers and children under 5 years, and to provide day nurseries.

1936 Public Health Act	Responsibilities of Local Authorities defined: sewage; drainage; removal of refuse; emission of excessive smoke; pure water supply; nuisances and offensive trades.
1942 Beveridge Report (Social Insurance and Allied Services)	Recommendations: The abolition of want 'through social insurance and by family needs'. To provide benefit for: unemployment; training; disability; retirement; medical treatment; funeral expenses; maternity. Provision of family allowances. Comprehensive health service.
1946 National Health Service Act	Free service by doctors and dentists. Hospital care and treatment. Drugs, medicines and appliances supplied free. Local Health Authorities duties: Health Committee; Health Centres; maternity, child welfare and midwifery services; ambulance services: home nursery service; the registration of nursing homes; health visitors; vaccination and immunisation; care and after-care of the sick; could provide day nurseries and home helps; local mental health service; care of the aged sick.
1956 Clean Air Act	Prohibited the emission of black smoke. Smokeless zones set up.
1960 Noise Abatement Act	Excessive noise prohibited.
1968 The Seebohm Report	Recommendations included: More to be done for the very young, the very old, the mentally and physically handicapped, disturbed adolescents. The establishment of local authority Social Services Departments to be responsible for: Children's welfare and guidance; mental health services; home help services; day nursery services; housing welfare services; services for the elderly.

	Department of Health and Social Security established.
1969 Local Government Social Services Act	Social Services Departments to be set up by Local Authorities.
1973 National Health Service Reorganisation Act	All health services unified under one authority to form the National Health Service, to come into force in April 1974.

NATIONAL HEALTH SERVICE (NHS)

The National Health Service started on 5th July 1948. While there are some variations in Scotland and Wales, the organisational structure is as follows:

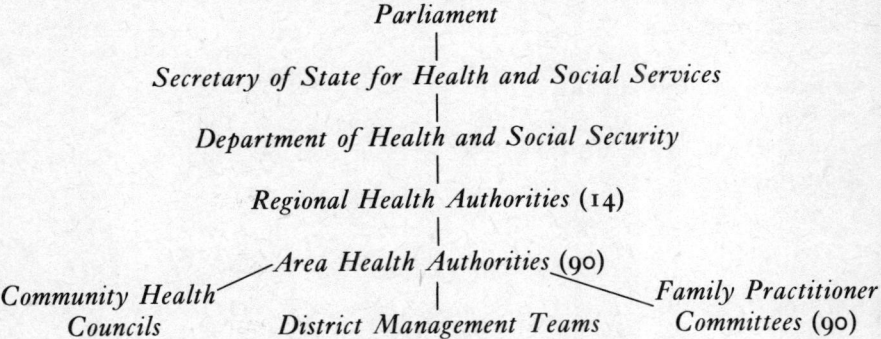

Parliament
|
Secretary of State for Health and Social Services
|
Department of Health and Social Security
|
Regional Health Authorities (14)
|
Area Health Authorities (90)

Community Health Councils   District Management Teams   Family Practitioner Committees (90)

Regional Health Authority
Responsible for the regional planning of all services.

Area Health Authority
Responsible for the provision of medical, dental, ophthalmic and phar-maceutical services.

District Management Team
Review the need for health care in the district.

Community Health Council
Represents the interests of the public in a Health District.

Family Practitioner Committee
Unifies the services of general practitioners.
Deals with disputes and complaints.

Health Service Commissioner (Ombudsman)
Has powers to investigate complaints from members of the public.

Finance
> General taxation over 85 per cent.
> National Insurance contributions approximately 9 per cent.
> Direct payments, e.g. prescriptions, dental and ophthalmic approximately 3 per cent.
> Proposals to change to an insurance based system are being considered.

HEALTH SERVICE

Available to everyone in UK and foreigners who become ill (under consideration). Free of charge except for:
a) Road traffic accidents.
b) Private accommodation or treatment in hospital, or extra amenities.
c) Drugs and appliances on prescription.
d) Dental treatment.
e) Spectacles.
Charges vary so find out the current charges.
Exemptions for some or all of the charges are made for the elderly, the chronically sick, expectant mothers, the needy, school children. (Check on current rules.)

PROVISIONS

a) *General Practitioner.* Everyone over the age of 16 may select a doctor from a list from the Family Practitioner Committee. If accepted, the person will be added to the doctor's list and issued with a medical card. Children are registered by their parent or guardian.
 A patient or a doctor may request a change through the Committee.
 In an emergency, treatment should be obtained from any NHS doctor.
b) *Hospital and Specialist Services.* Patients are normally referred by their general practitioner except for emergency treatment.
c) *Drugs and Dressings (Prescriptions).* There is a payment for each article. Refer to above.
d) *Dental Service.* There is freedom to consult any NHS dentist. Treatment is free for school children, expectant mothers and for those on Supplementary Benefit or Family Income Supplement.
e) *Ophthalmic Service.* Sight testing is free but there is a charge for spectacles, with exemption for school children and those on a low income.
f) *Appliances*, e.g. artificial limbs, hearing aids, may be obtained.

g) *Vaccination and immunisation* for young children, people travelling abroad, or in case of an epidemic or possible contact.
h) *Maternal and Child Health Services* (*Refer Modules 2 and 3*)
i) *Family planning* (*Refer Module 2*)
j) *Health visiting* for the ill, elderly, young children, expectant and nursing mothers.
k) *Services for the elderly and disabled.* Health visitors. Home nursing. Day hospitals. (Social Services supply home helps, meals on wheels, day centres, library service, etc. – with voluntary organisations.)
l) *School Health Service.* Medical, dental, eye and head inspections.
m) *Services for the mentally handicapped.* Hospital services and some assessment facilities.
n) *Sexually transmitted diseases.* Treatment is free and confidential. Referral can be through a GP or by the patient.
o) *Abortion* (*Refer Module 2*)
p) *Drug addiction.* Treatment for narcotic drug dependence and for alcoholism is provided on an out-patient basis but sometimes there is in-patient treatment for particular problems.
q) *Blood bank.* The blood donor system is an important contribution to the NHS.

THE NATIONAL HEALTH SERVICE AND THE PUBLIC

The facilities offered to the public by the Health Service, and the opportunities available to achieve the best possible physical and mental health, are dependent for their success on the co-operation of individuals and families.

HEALTH

The definition of health by the World Health Organisation, given at the beginning of this module, is 'A state of complete physical, mental and social well-being and not simply the absence of disease or infirmity'. However, people may have a physical defect and yet be healthy. During illness there is usually an attempt to obtain treatment but when illness is over, health may be forgotten or even neglected. Health is not just a freedom from illness. There should be a positive approach to health. People should be aware of how they can help themselves to try to ensure good health; how families and friends can help each other; what facilities are available through the community. It could be concluded, after a study of the structure of the NHS, that there appears to be ample provision in the UK for all aspects of health, yet there are a number of problems still in existence. People still suffer and die from diseases. Children are neglected, in simple matters such as the care of teeth, or in much more serious ways, e.g. child cruelty. There is much self-abuse of health, e.g. drug-taking, smoking, obesity, neglect of symptoms which lead to physical and mental illness. Individuals and families must be made aware of the importance of a positive approach to physical and mental health for themselves, and should appreciate that they are responsible for community health through national and local government.

Body health and efficient functioning

Knowledge of the structure of the body and its functioning will provide information which should help in a positive approach to health. (*Refer to a book on human biology*) (*Refer to this module for Principles of Health Care, p. 65*)

HEALTH HAZARDS

INFECTIOUS DISEASES

Infectious diseases are caused by pathogenic viruses, bacteria, or other micro-organisms entering the body and causing infection.

a) *Viruses*. Different viruses cause chicken pox; the common cold; influenza; measles; German measles; poliomyelitis, etc. Viruses may damage the body cells permanently, e.g. poliomyelitis.

b) *Bacteria* reproduce rapidly if given suitable conditions of food, warmth, moisture and time. Not all cause disease (are pathogenic); some are used in cheese making and in brewing, etc. Pathogenic bacteria cause boils; cholera; diphtheria; food poisoning, etc. They can form toxins which are resistant to high temperatures and this is particularly dangerous if contaminated food is stored and reheated.

c) *Fungi* can cause infections of the skin, e.g. ringworm; athlete's foot.

d) *Animal parasites*, e.g. scabies, mites and intestinal worms.

e) *Protozoa* are simple one-cell animals, e.g. amoebae, causing amoebic dysentery.

Infection occurs when the organisms, having entered the body, multiply and cause symptoms according to the particular disease – rash; cough; sore throat; pain; raised temperature; loss of appetite, etc., and then damage the body according to the type of disease and the degree of infection.

Pathogenic organisms enter the body by swallowing, breathing in (nose or mouth) or penetrating the skin.

Direct infection can be caused by:
a) droplet infection from the spray of moisture when an infected person coughs, sneezes or speaks;
b) droplets from infected faeces and urine;
c) contact with infected skin or body organs.

Indirect infection can be caused by:
a) flies, mice, rats, cockroaches, etc. which carry pathogenic organisms and contaminate food;
b) insects which carry organisms of disease and transmit these by injection (bites);
c) hands which have become infected by pathogenic organisms can pass infection to the person concerned or can contaminate others;
d) carriers, who not apparently ill, can carry pathogenic organisms in the bowels, throat or nose, and infect others;
e) food which is contaminated at source, e.g. an infected animal, or becomes infected by handling;
f) water contaminated by sewage or other decaying animal matter.

Principles of care

a) Knowledge of how disease is caused, the symptoms and when to seek help.
b) Preventive measures – sound nutrition; personal hygiene; exercise and fresh air; care of babies, children and the elderly; hygiene in the home; hygiene in the community.
c) Defences against infection – immunity; vaccination.

Sexually transmitted diseases

Diseases of the genital tract which can be passed on by sexual contact. Included are: venereal diseases; urethritis; herpes.

Principles of care

a) Avoid promiscuity.
b) Seek help if any possible symptoms develop.
c) Seek help if a sexual partner develops a disease or symptoms.
NHS Clinics provide confidential checks and treatment.

FUNCTIONAL DISEASES

There are a number of diseases which are caused by malfunction of body systems, tissues or cells, or hormone imbalance.

a) *Heart disease*

   Heart disease (cardio-vascular disease) is directly responsible for 40 per cent of all deaths in UK. There has been a rapid increase over the last 30 years. Although the causes have not been scientifically proved, doctors consider that a style of living could be responsible:

   (i) *Stress*, e.g. worry about job security; keeping up standards of living.
   (ii) *Lack of exercise* caused by increased use of cars; spectator sports; watching television.
   (iii) *Malnutrition*. Obesity (excess weight) increases the work of the cardiac system. Possibly the intake of saturated fats. (*Refer Module 9*)
   (iv) *Smoking* is considered to double the risk of heart disease.

b) *Cancers*

   The causes of cancers (malignant growths) are not yet fully known. Can generally be cured provided that early specialist help is obtained.

c) *Rheumatism and arthritis*

   Diseases of the nerves, muscles, bones and joints which are considered to be functional diseases but may be caused by a deficiency in the diet.

DEFICIENCY DISEASES

Caused by a lack of one or more nutrients, e.g. anaemia is caused particularly by a lack of iron but there may also be a deficiency of vitamins of the B group and A and C. It is difficult to separate deficiency diseases from functional diseases as the problem may arise from the inability of the body to utilise particular nutrients although the supply is adequate. Malnutrition or under-nutrition may be responsible. (*Refer Module 9*)

Obesity is not strictly a deficiency disease but it is a form of malnutrition. (*Refer Module 9*)

Anorexia nervosa is self-inflicted under-nutrition by self-starvation which sometimes occurs in adolescents, usually in girls, as a reaction against 'puppy fat' or as the result of an emotional upset, disappointment in love, or a bereavement. The intake of food is cut down to an inadequate level. Supervision can result in food being secretly disposed of or vomited. Prolonged starvation causes damage to body organs, particularly in the digestive system, extreme thinness, and possibly death.

HANDICAP

a) *Physical handicap*

Disabilities may have happened at birth, be the results of an accident or the effects of a disease. There is a need to identify ways in which disabilities can be overcome whenever possible, and to try to understand the problems. Facilities are provided by the Health, Social and Education Services.

b) *Mental handicap*

May be caused by birth damage, an accident, the effects of a disease or be inherited. There is a double problem when there is both physical and mental handicap. The families involved have many responsibilities and need all the support possible from the Health, Social and Education Services.

c) *Mental illness*

May be minor and of short duration or can be very serious. Specialist help is necessary when there are signs of stress, e.g. depression, withdrawal, aggression, over-anxiety, etc.

d) *Social handicap/disadvantage*

Is not related to any social class. It could result from:

 (i) living conditions which are not adequate regarding food, shelter and clothing, or are unhygienic;

 (ii) physical damage – accidents, disease, cruelty, e.g. battered baby;

 (iii) emotional deprivation – lack of love and security;

 (iv) intellectual deprivation – inability to communicate in writing, language or reading. May be a cultural problem.

A family may have few financial problems but the children may suffer from one or more of the above problems which can result in physical or emotional damage, misery and an inability to take advantage of educational facilities. The Health, Social and Education Services will provide help.

The public has a responsibility to identify cases of child neglect or cruelty.

DRUGS

Not usually harmful if taken under medical supervision in recommended doses. **N.B.** the drug 'thalidomide' did cause damage to unborn babies. However, drugs can produce harmful side effects if taken in excess. Constant use can lead to dependency.

The over-use and dependence on drugs can lead to: death; serious damage to the body; impaired body functions; coma; personality changes; irresponsible actions; hallucinations; depression; violence.

The terms 'hard' and 'soft' drugs are misleading.

ALL DRUGS ARE POTENTIALLY DANGEROUS.

The misuse of household chemicals is harmful, e.g. glue-sniffing. The liver, kidneys and nervous system can be damaged and there can be unconsciousness and possibly death.

Drugs in pregnancy. (*Refer Module 2*)

ALCOHOL

Alcohol is one of the most common drugs. Alcoholism, dependency on the drug, is on the increase for both men and women. The consumption of alcohol in the UK is estimated by a recent survey to have risen by over 90 per cent between 1970 and 1980.

Alcohol can:
a) slow down reactions and cloud judgement so causing accidents in the home and on the road;
b) impair efficiency and performance at work;
c) harm body organs, particularly the liver, and lead to severe illness and death;
d) cause excessive weight;
e) damage surface blood vessels;
f) cause unpleasant after effects – 'hangover';
g) lead to financial problems for the drinker and the family;
h) cause family disputes and crises;
i) affect foetal development. (*Refer Module 2*)

Alcoholics Anonymous provides guidance and support for the alcoholic and the family. The Health Service offers treatment. It is against the law to sell alcoholic drinks to people under the age of 18 years.

TOBACCO SMOKING

Smoke from tobacco is thought to be a contributory factor to bronchitis, coronary thrombosis, sinusitus, laryngitis and to aggravate conditions such as gastric ulcers, as well as the danger of lung cancer. Smoke not only damages the smoker's body, but exposes others to danger. Smoking in pregnancy is harmful to the foetus (*Refer Module 2*). A heavy concentration of smoke in a room causes non-smokers to inhale as much carbon monoxide as if they had smoked a cigarette (passive smoking). Children living in an atmosphere contaminated by smoke tend to suffer from certain respiratory diseases. People with respiratory diseases have aggravation from smoke.

In 1957, the Medical Research Council of Great Britain published findings upon the relationship of cigarette smoking to lung cancer. Since then the Government has mounted campaigns against smoking: the advertising of cigarettes on television was prohibited in 1965; since 1971, cigarette packets have to contain a Government warning that cigarettes can seriously damage health; in 1973 figures for tar and nicotine content in various brands were published by the Government and advertisements for cigarettes now contain a statement about the level; by-laws allow local authorities to restrict smoking in public places.

There have been efforts to prevent the habit of smoking among children. It is illegal to serve tobacco to people under the age of 16 years. Department stores and other public buildings contain *No Smoking* notices, on the grounds of public safety as well as public health.

The habit of smoking may be difficult to stop and many people seek help from doctors or anti-smoking clinics.

POLLUTION

Despite the Clean Air Act 1955, pollution by smoke still exists, and now there are perhaps more dangerous forms of pollution.

a) *Air Pollution*
   The amount of carbon monoxide and lead has increased because of the number of motor vehicles. The development of new processes in industry and in the generation of power has led to the further emission of chemicals and new health hazards. (*Refer to Pesticides, p. 62 and Module 9*)
b) *Industrial Waste*
   Industrial development has resulted in the increase of industrial waste.

Some of the waste is dangerous to man, animals and vegetation. There are many problems in disposal:

Waste tips – dangerous chemicals have been dumped on tips which can be reached by children.

Sewerage systems – industrial waste products and detergent foam have caused problems. **Note:** modern detergents do not cause excessive foaming.

Water supply – industrial waste products and detergents cause problems.

N.B. The disposal of nuclear waste causes particular problems.

c) *Sewage*

This country has a complex system of sewerage but there are still rural areas where sewage may seep into, and pollute, sources of water. It should be noted that sewerage systems in many large cities have been in existence for well over a century and are in need of repair.

d) *Pesticides/herbicides*

The increasing use of pesticides in agriculture, particularly spraying from the air, is causing concern. Contamination to birds, insects, animals and vegetation has resulted but it is difficult to identify any harm to man. However, some sprays are now forbidden, e.g. DDT. (*Refer Module 9*)

e) *Noise*

There is concern about the increased amount of noise which can be considered as a form of pollution. Excessive loud noise – in certain industries, discos or pop concerts – could damage hearing. Exposure to noise can add to stress which may only cause irritation or emotional upset, but could be a contributory factor in heart disease and mental illness. (*Refer Book 2 – The Home*)

ACCIDENTS
(*Refer also to 'O' Level Cookery*)

An accident has been defined as an 'unforseen event' or a 'chance occurrence' but most accidents are preventable. Accidents occur in the community or at work, but the highest percentage occurs in the home.

HOME ACCIDENTS

Home accidents include falls resulting in breaks, fractures, brain damage; burns and scalds; cuts; poisoning; suffocation; electric shock.

Principles of care

a) Try to ensure that the home is hazard free. Encourage the use of safe practices for tools and equipment.

b) Pay particular attention to the safety of babies, young children (note the danger in some toys), the ill, the mentally and physically handicapped, the elderly.

c) Store household materials, chemicals, drugs, plastic bags, and tools and equipment which could be dangerous, in a safe place.

d) Follow instructions for any piece of equipment and never use in an unsafe condition. Note the danger of trailing flexes. Use a fire guard where there are babies, children and old people.

e) Have installations and repairs done by qualified staff, especially for electricity and gas.

f) Avoid slippery floors, loose rugs and carpets, especially on stairs.

g) Learn First Aid. Have an adequate First Aid Box.

h) Have the doctor's telephone number available. Train children to use the telephone and instruct them how to call help.

i) Insure against accidents in the home and garden for the family, visitors and workmen.

ACCIDENTS IN THE COMMUNITY

Include road accidents (which are on the increase); falls; drowning; suffocation; burns.

Principles of care

a) Take action against dangerous areas in the environment. Help the young, elderly and handicapped.

b) Never drive under the influence of drink or drugs (a criminal offence).

c) Never drive unless qualified and obey the driving laws – licence; roadworthy vehicle; insurance (criminal offences). Pedestrians must also obey the rules of the road.

d) Never take a boat out unless you can control it safely. Learn to swim and do not swim in hazardous conditions.

e) Do not engage in sports such as rock climbing or pot-holing, unless you are experienced or with an expert guide. The route and estimated time of arrival should be reported before departure.

f) Wear protective clothing for sports, driving a motor bike, etc.

g) Try not to smoke in public places – this may be prohibited. Extinguish cigarettes safely.
h) Seek specialist help in the case of an accident. If necessary ring 999, giving clear instructions as to the location of the accident and the service required. Make the injured comfortable and give First Aid, unless there is a danger of further injury.

ACCIDENTS AT WORK

Places of work are protected by Safety Laws. Firms have safety committees but people put themselves in danger by unsafe practices.

Accidents at work include falls; cuts; breaks and fractures; burns and scalds; facial injuries especially to the eyes; scalp injuries.

Principles of care

a) Follow safety regulations; use safety guards; wear protective clothing.
b) Report any broken or dangerous equipment or hazards.
c) Do not smoke in restricted areas. See that cigarettes are properly extinguished.
d) Wipe up spilled liquids, especially chemicals.
e) Do not resort to unsafe practices or irresponsible behaviour, e.g. drinking on duty.
f) Report any accidents. Follow the required procedure.
g) Ensure that accident cases receive specialist care. Use First Aid until help can be obtained.

FIRST AID

First Aid is mainly preventative and should not be considered to be the final treatment of accidents except for minor damage – small cut, etc. If in doubt seek help.

Emergency measures include:
a) Stemming the flow of blood from a vein or artery.
b) Covering burns or scalds with a clean, dry cloth.
c) After a serious fall, not moving the patient but providing comfort and warmth.

d) Switching off the current before touching a person who has suffered an electric shock.

Do not attempt any treatment unless qualified to do so. Send for the doctor or telephone 999 for the emergency service required.

It is possible to obtain training in First Aid from the St John Ambulance Association or the British Red Cross Society.

FIRST AID BOX

Keep readily available, but out of the reach of young children. Stock with sterile bandages, cotton wool, lint, adhesive plaster, antiseptic, scissors.

PRINCIPLES OF HEALTH CARE

Being healthy involves body care and maintenance, and an awareness of health hazards. Principles of health care are the responsibility of the individual, the family or group, and the community.

HEALTH AND THE INDIVIDUAL

The individual should assume certain responsibilities for health as early in life as possible. Much will depend upon habits which are established. (*Refer Modules 3 and 4*)

PERSONAL HYGIENE

This is important, not only for the prevention of disease, but is necessary to prevent offensive body odours, poor skin, lank hair and dirty nails.
a) The body should be washed every day and dried thoroughly.
b) Deodorants/anti-perspirants help to prevent odour if used on a clean skin and if the instructions are followed.
c) Talcum powder helps to dry and perfume the skin but does not prevent body odour and neither does perfume itself.
d) Hygiene during menstruation is most important.
e) Rules of hygiene should be followed during illness.

Particular attention should be given to the following:

EYES

The sensation of light is received by nerve cells in the retina and passed through nerve fibres to the optic nerve and to the brain. Rays of light are focused on retinal cells by means of a lens behind the cornea. The iris regulates the amount of light passed through and also gives colour to the eye.

Protection is provided by:
a) fluid (vitreous humour) in the eye;
b) an outer covering which forms a transparent cornea;
c) conjunctiva which lines the eyelids;
d) eyelids and eyelashes;
e) tears.

Tears are secreted from the lacrimal glands, and contain a small amount of sodium chloride. They normally drain into the nose after passing across the eyes.

The functions of tears are to moisten the eyes, to provide a slight anti-septic, to remove dust and foreign bodies and to indicate emotion or pain.

THE EYE

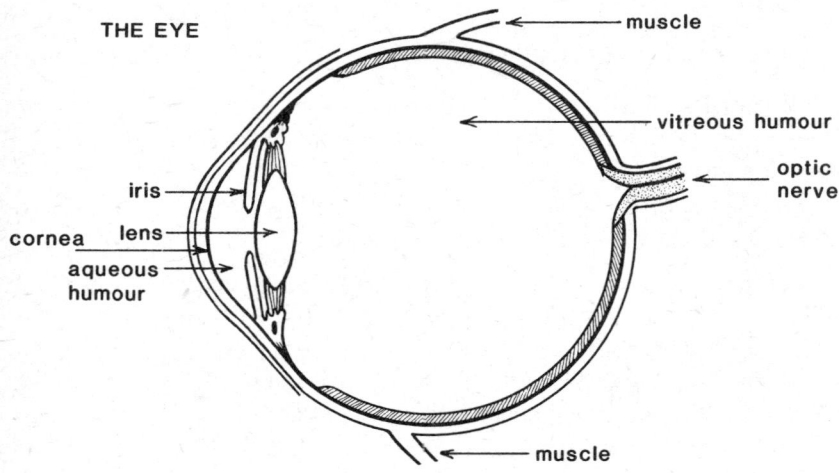

Principles of care
a) Balanced diet with an adequate supply of vitamin A.
b) Cleanliness. No rubbing or poking. Care with eye make-up.

c) Avoidance of strain, close work in poor light, or prolonged sessions in bright sunshine or other strong light.

d) Specialist help for changes in vision or difficulty in seeing; squinting; frowning; screwing-up eyes; watery or red eyes.

e) Spectacles should be worn if prescribed by an optician. The excessive use of sunglasses is not good for the eyes.

EARS

The ear is an organ which perceives sensations of sound and enables body balance.

Outer ear conducts sound waves to the membrane of the ear drum which vibrates.

Middle ear contains three small bones which pick up the vibrations, alter the intensity, and conduct the sound to another membrane which communicates with the inner ear.

Inner ear – a shell-like structure called the cochlea which converts sound waves into impulses which are passed on to the brain. The inner ear also

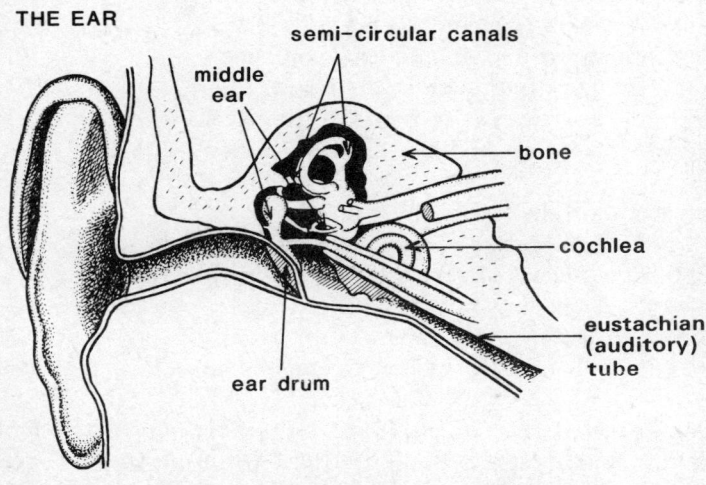

THE EAR

contains the semicircular canals which aid balance. Fluid in the canals moves as the head is moved and this indicates whether the body is upright and in which direction the head is turned.

Eustachian tube – a passage connecting the middle ear to the throat. When suffering from a cold, this passage may become blocked so that there is a lack of sensitivity to vibrations and so, a temporary deafness. The tube is also affected when going up to, or down from, a height.

Principles of care

a) Balanced diet.
b) Cleanliness. No poking of the ears. No excess liquid down the ears.
c) Avoidance of very loud, continuous noise.
d) Specialist help for any hearing difficulty, noise or pain in the ear, a discharging ear or any severe blow on the ear.

TEETH

Temporary (deciduous) teeth form as cartilage by about the fourth month of pregnancy. At birth, the process of calcification has begun, and the 20 deciduous teeth are usually complete by about $2\frac{1}{2}$ years and begin to loosen by about 5 years.

Permanent (second) teeth erupt at about 5 years.
a) There should be 32 permanent teeth.
b) The top and bottom sets should each contain:
    4 incisors (sharp cutting teeth at the front);
    2 canine (grasping teeth at each side of the incisors);
    4 pre-molars (grinding teeth);
    6 molars;
    Wisdom teeth are the last of the molars.
Each tooth is in three parts – crown; root; neck. Inside each tooth is pulp which contains the nerve. The outside of a tooth is dentine which is covered on the crown with enamel. Enamel is the hardest body substance but it is never regenerated, so once it is damaged, decay begins to occur. Teeth are set into sockets, supported by ligaments and the tooth base is protected by the gums.

Dental decay (dental caries) is the destruction of the fabric of a tooth as a result of acid formed by the action of bacteria (from plaque) on sugar. It is

STRUCTURE OF A TOOTH

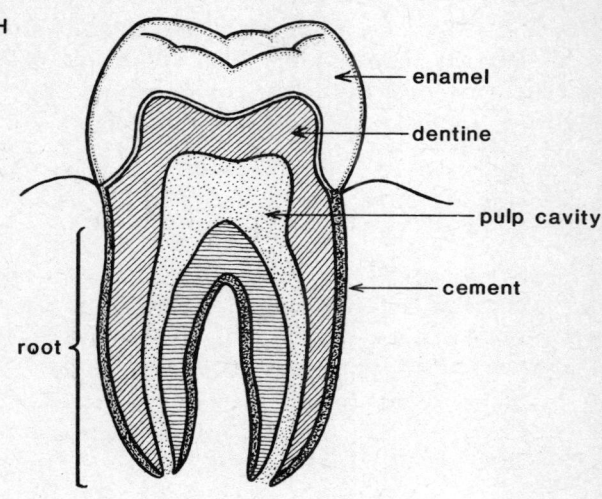

enamel

dentine

pulp cavity

cement

root

TEETH

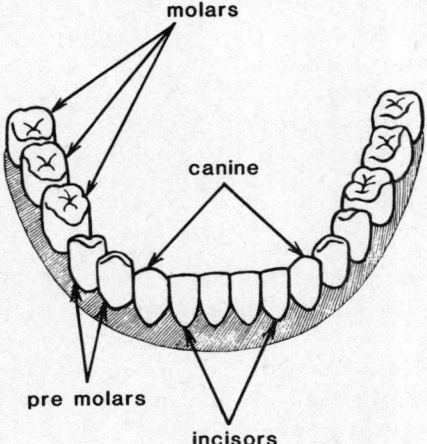

molars

canine

pre molars

incisors

not the amount of sugar consumed which is significant, as the length of time it remains in the mouth and on the teeth without being cleaned off, but obviously the more sugar which is eaten, the more this is likely to remain and be converted into acid.

Plaque is formed from bacteria in the mouth which adhere to the surface of teeth. Regular, thorough, brushing will remove plaque and so help to prevent the decay of teeth caused by the formation of acid from sugar. Disclosing tablets will indicate the presence of plaque.

Periodontal disease is the breakdown of gum and supporting bone which causes the loosening of teeth and gum disease. A contributory factor is the presence of plaque left on the teeth.

Surveys have shown that in the UK:
95 per cent of children in the 5–14 year age group are in the first stages of periodontal disease. 37 per cent of people over 16 years have no teeth of their own (44 per cent in Scotland).

Principles of care

a) A diet with a restricted sugar intake – sugar itself, sweets, and cakes, biscuits, puddings and cereals containing sugar.
b) A balanced diet with sufficient calcium, protein and vitamins C and D.
c) Knowledge about the reasons for, and the prevention of, tooth decay and gum disease.
d) A regular pattern of dental care:
   (i) Use the right size and shape of brush to reach all surfaces. After about 3 months use, replace a brush.
   (ii) A mild toothpaste will aid cleaning but it is the brushing which is important. Fluoride in toothpaste may help against the establishment of plaque.
   (iii) Brush the teeth up and down, back and front, and brush over the gums. Brushing should continue for at least 3 minutes. Brush before going to bed and, if possible, after each meal, snack, or the eating of sweets.
   (iv) Dental floss can be used to clean between the teeth.
   (v) Visit the dentist regularly for an inspection and cleaning, every 6 months at least, for attention to any aching or loose teeth or bleeding gums; for misshapen teeth.

SKIN

The skin is the outer covering of the body and is composed of:

The epidermis (outer layer) which is a protective surface of flattened cells composed of keratin.

The dermis (inner layer) which contains sweat glands, sebaceous glands, nerve fibres, blood vessels and capillaries and hair follicles.

a) *Sweat glands*

Sweat glands are found all over the body but in particular on the forehead, arm pits, palms and the soles of the feet. Sweat (perspiration) which filters out through the sweat glands is mainly water with minute quantities of salts, mainly sodium chloride, and other waste products from the blood. There is constant secretion of sweat which evaporates quickly and is not observed (insensible sweat). When the body is warm or under stress, the sweat is heavier and observable (sensible sweat). The more sweat which is produced, the less urine is excreted and vice versa. **N.B.** Because sodium chloride (salt) is excreted in sweat, an extra salt supply may be necessary for people in hot climates or working under hot conditions. The skin plays an important part in the regulation of body temperature. It draws heat from the body during evaporation.

b) *Sebaceous glands*

The glands form a greasy secretion called sebum which helps to keep the skin supple and the hair from becoming dry. Over-production of sebum or failure to remove by washing will (usually) result in greasy skin and hair.

Principles of care

a) Balanced diet with an adequate supply of vitamins C and A.

b) Rashes, bruises without a known reason, or growths on the skin may be symptoms of disease, a nervous illness or malnutrition. Seek specialist help.

c) Minor cuts should stop bleeding by blood clotting, but serious cuts need medical attention. **N.B.** haemophilia.

d) Sweat and sebum which are allowed to stay on the body collect dirt, smell unpleasant, and provide an ideal medium for the growth of bacteria and the development of diseases. Regular washing is necessary.

e) Excessive exposure to the sun can cause the skin to burn and leads to dryness and wrinkles (and possibly skin cancer). Strong detergents can dry and irritate the skin.

HAIR AND SKIN STRUCTURE

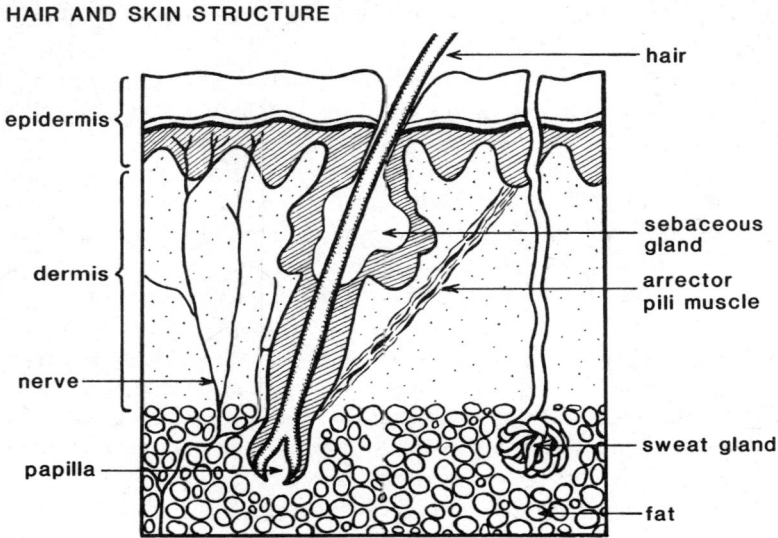

HAIR

Hair develops in the hair follicles and the whole surface of the body is covered with hair although much is practically invisible. Most of the hair (between 100,000 and 200,000 hairs) is on the scalp. The length of hair varies according to the person and the age of the hair. A healthy hair drops out after about 3 years. Heredity is usually responsible for baldness in men and there is little chance of regrowth. *Head lice* breed in hair and can be passed from one head to another. Children's hair in particular should be inspected regularly, combed and brushed daily, and washed as necessary. If head lice are discovered, a special soap or shampoo can be obtained.

Principles of care

a) Balanced diet – an excess of fat can make hair greasy.
b) Hair can be damaged by – alkaline shampoos; excessive sunlight; over

bleaching or colouring; back combing; tight plaiting; strong permanent waving. Dandruff, flakes of dry skin or oxidised sebum needs to be treated.

c) Avoid conditions which could cause damage. Comb and brush hair regularly, avoiding combs with sharp teeth and brushes with sharp bristles. Wash regularly. Conditioners should be used according to hair type and instructions followed.

d) Seek specialist help for any rash, persistant irritation or hair falling out.

NAILS

Nails are outgrowths of the skin and are composed of a closely packed mass of keratin. An average nail grows about 0.3 cm each month. If the nail bed is damaged, the new nail may be misshapen. Brittle or splitting nails may be caused by: alkaline substances; poor health; malnutrition; careless manicuring; over-use of nail varnish or remover.

Biting nails is an unpleasant, disfiguring habit. Encouragement to break the habit or painting the nails with a bitter substance may help. Nails which are not kept clean not only look unsightly, but they may harbour bacteria.

Principles of care

a) Balanced diet with sufficient calcium and vitamins D and C.
b) Regular cutting and careful manicuring.

FEET

The health and comfort of feet are affected by: the weight of the body; posture; correct or ill-fitting shoes; shoes with too high a heel or giving too little support; plastic shoes and nylon tights or socks.

Sweat glands are plentiful upon the soles of the feet, so this, together with the feet becoming over-heated by being enclosed for long periods, causes a lot of sweat to be produced. Stale sweat smells unpleasant and provides a place for the growth of micro-organisms and resultant diseases, e.g. Athlete's foot.

Principles of care

a) Wash feet regularly and dry thoroughly.

b) Wear shoes which fit correctly and support the weight of the body.
c) Do not wear man-made materials, e.g. plastic or nylon, for long periods.
d) Seek specialist help for corns, callouses, broken skin.

PERSONAL FITNESS

a) A balanced diet is needed to keep the body in condition and to enable efficient functioning. (*Refer 'O' Level Cookery*)
b) Fresh air and sunshine are necessary to keep the body healthy.
c) Exercise is necessary for body development and functioning, to keep the body supple and in good shape. It should be taken by people of all ages and all conditions provided that any specialist advice is followed. Limited, regular exercise is better than spurts of violent activity. Exercise can be provided by active and not spectator sports, walking or cycling (instead of riding in a car), housework, gardening and manual work and activities of all kinds.
d) Body posture is most important.
e) Sleep and rest are necessary for the avoidance of stress, to allow body systems to relax and, it is now considered, to provide opportunities for the brain to deal with an accumulation of information. The amount of sleep needed is usually 7 to 8 hours for an adult. Babies and children need more sleep and old people may need less. If regular sleep is not possible, even though the conditions are satisfactory – comfort, warmth and quietness – a doctor should be consulted.
f) Social relationships with people of all ages, but particularly one's own age group (peer group), are important for a happy, balanced life.
g) Leisure activities – sport, reading, music, dancing, hobbies, etc., add variety to life and make a more interesting, less stressful life.
h) Intellectual activities – reading, study, discussion, music, aid full personal development.
i) Drugs can harm the body and should be avoided unless prescribed. (*Refer to p. 60*)
j) Specialist help should be sought for any symptoms of ill health or body malfunctioning, and the advice given should be followed.

HEALTH AND THE FAMILY

Members of a family (or a group of people) have responsibilities for health which are individual and communal. Each member should assume some degree of personal responsibility early in life. Parents have to make decisions for their children and educate them towards desirable health habits. A sound relationship should be established with the family doctor. and knowledge should be obtained about other specialist help – clinics and advice centres, dentists, opticians and hospitals. (*Refer Modules 2, 3, 4 and 5*)

HEALTH AND THE COMMUNITY

All families and individual members of a community should play their part in trying to create a community which is a healthy and pleasant place in which to live. People need to involve themselves in communal activities. There needs to be an oversight of local and national planning for building roads, industries, shops, houses, etc., and an awareness of the dangers of pollution – in air, water, sewage, refuse and noise. There should be a concern for those people in need of care.

MODULE SIX REFERENCES

Health Education Council (for England, Wales, Northern Ireland)
78 New Oxford Street
London WC1A 1AH

Scottish Health Education Unit
Health Education Centre
21 Landsdowne Crescent
Edinburgh EH12 5EH

Royal Society for the Prevention of Accidents (ROSPA)
6 Buckingham Place
London SW1E 6HR

British Standards Institution
2 Park Street
London W1A 2BS

Central Council for the Disabled
34 Eccleston Square
London SW1V 1PE

ASH (Action on Smoking and Health)
Margaret Pyke Centre
27–35 Mortimer Street
London W1A 4QW

General Dental Council
37 Wimpole Street
London W1M 8DQ

Eye Care Information Bureau
55 Park Lane
London W1

National Association for Maternal and Child Welfare
1 South Audley Street
London W1

Area Health Authority
(Obtain local address)

St John Ambulance Association
1 Grosvenor Crescent
London SW1

British Red Cross Society
(Obtain local address)

Children's Foot Health Register
9 Sir Thomas Street
London SE1 9SA

Town and Country Planning
   Association
Environmental Education Unit
17 Carlton House Terrace
London SW1Y 5AS

Teachers' Advisory Council on
   Alcohol and Drug addiction
437 Royal Exchange
Manchester M2 7EP

Books

Visual Human Biology G. D. Chalk and G. P. J. Baster (Edward Arnold)

FOLLOW-UP ACTIVITIES

1. Draw up a routine of personal care for a child of 10 years and a routine for yourself.
2. Compare the provision for community health in 1850 and in 1982.
3. Consider the possible dangers in a kitchen and suggest how the dangers could be overcome.
4. Investigate the work of an individual who has contributed to health reform.
5. Find out about the present provisions of the National Health Service and list charges and exemptions.
6. Investigate a 'health hazard' and list the dangers and the steps to be taken to avoid the hazard.
7. Consider preventative health care for: a) a child of 2 years; b) an elderly person.

FINANCE

MONEY

The organisation of personal or family finance is important. Money is of little value in itself. In the past, gold and silver were used to make coins but now money is made from paper and cheaper metals. The value of money lies in its purchasing power which is guaranteed by a government. (Read the statement on a banknote.) Before the development of money there was bartering and exchange of goods and services. Money evolved as a convenient way of measuring value.

WAGES/SALARY

Money is received in the form of wages or salary, income from savings or investment, from a pension or allowance, or as a gift. A pay slip (the statement of wages or salary) should indicate the amount earned monthly or weekly, the deductions, and the amount of money which is actually received by the worker.

Terms concerned with payment for work and deductions are as follows:

Money is a measure of the value of goods or services.

Wage is a sum paid for work each week and is usually based on hourly rates for the work.

Salary is a sum paid for work which is usually stated as an annual amount and paid at monthly intervals.

Overtime is payment for work beyond the normal working hours. There is usually a fixed rate of payment.

Piece-work is payment for work by fixing a rate for a work process and paying according to the number of processes completed.

Bonus is an additional payment to wages for a particular event, e.g. Christmas, or for a particular effort to finish a job, etc.

Fringe benefits are received in addition to a wage or salary and may include a car, a house, etc. They are required to be declared for income tax.

Gross wage or salary is before deductions of tax, National Insurance, etc.

Net wage or salary is the sum remaining after deductions, i.e. the sum actually received.

Income tax is a sum levied by the Government on the income received by an individual or a married couple.

PAYE (Pay As You Earn) is a sum deducted from wages or salary to cover the estimated income tax.

National Insurance contribution is the sum paid by an employee towards the services provided by the National Health and Social Security Departments. (The employer also pays a contribution.)

Superannuation/Pension contribution is a sum paid towards a pension from a place of work on retirement.

Trade Union is an organisation of workers engaged in the same trade or occupation. It is formed for the purpose of improving conditions of work and pay. Dues are paid by the members and may be based on the amount earned.

THE INCOME AND EXPENDITURE OF THE COUNTRY

A country needs a supply of money to take care of its people, to provide social security, law and order, health, defence, education, roads, agriculture, civil service, etc. Money comes from taxes on people and property, and from natural assets, e.g. oil. The Chancellor of the Exchequer draws up a Budget each March/April, and at other times as necessary. In the Budget, the allocation of money for the needs of the country and details of any taxes are indicated to Parliament and to the public. Some taxes are levied (the direction and collection of a tax) at local government level, e.g. rates.

INCOME TAX

This tax is applied to income which is received as a wage or salary or from other sources such as interest from a bank account. The income tax year runs from 6th April to the following 5th April (the Financial Year). Income tax forms are sent and have to be completed, giving the information required. (*Refer to a form for the current year*)

INCOME: Year ended 5 April 1981

	See Note	Details	Amount for year	
			Self £	Wife £
EARNINGS		Own full-time employment. *You need not enter details or pay relating to your own full-time employment but you must enter tips below.*		
	1	Wife's employment *Employer's name and address Works No. (if any)*		
	2	All other earnings *Type of work*		
		Name and address of anyone for whom work done		
	3	Tips and incidental receipts from ALL sources		
		If you or your wife received a taxed sum from trustees of an approved profit sharing scheme *tick "√" here* ▶	*(see also note 31)*	
		If the duties of your employment were performed wholly or partly outside the United Kingdom *tick "√" here* ▶		
		Expenses against earnings	Self £	Wife £
	4	*If a fixed deduction applies tick "√" here* ▶ [Self │ Wife]		
		Where no fixed deduction applies state nature and amounts of expenses		
	5	Fees or subscriptions to professional bodies *Name of professional body*		
SOCIAL SECURITY PENSIONS AND BENEFITS	6	Retirement pension or Old Person's pension *If wife's pension paid as a result of her own contributions tick "√" here to claim wife's earned income allowance* ▶		
	7	Widow's and other benefits *Nature of benefit* .... *(See identity page of Order Book)*		
OTHER PENSIONS	8	*Payer's name Address* Pensions from former employers and other pensions		

Part of a specimen income tax form. © Crown copyright.

a) Income received – from employment; bank deposits and investments; fringe benefits; other sources.
b) Allowances claimed – dependent relatives; handicap; housekeeper's services; age; son's or daughter's services; payment for tools, etc. Personal allowances are indicated by the tax office and are at a fixed rate. (*Refer to current year*)

If forms are not returned by the date indicated, full tax will usually be charged (without the deduction of allowances).

All people are required by law to pay tax from the time they are born if there is sufficient income. People below the income level for the payment of tax still have to complete a form but no tax will be charged. Help in completing forms can be obtained from some banks or from the social services.

Tax does not have to be paid on: interest on savings certificates; Social Security or Unemployment benefits; building society interest. (Check current regulations.)

Notice of coding

This is a form which is sent to the tax payer. It indicates allowances which have been given against income. The tax code is stated. (*Refer to leaflet P3 from the tax office*)

Appeals

If there is disagreement with the tax assessment, an appeal may be made to the inspector of taxes within 30 days (*Refer to leaflet 64D*). The inspector may agree to an amendment of the assessment. If there is no agreement the appeal can be taken to the General Commissioners, an independent body.

Interest is charged on tax paid late. In the case of an appeal, interest is usually payable 30 days after the date of appeal.

Prosecution for non-payment of tax. If tax is levied, this must be paid or there will be a prosecution.

Deduction of tax

Employed persons – notice of coding is sent to the employer who will deduct tax through PAYE each week or month.

Self-employed persons – direction for payment is made by the tax collector.

Rates of tax

Rates are fixed by the Chancellor. There is a percentage rate on income which increases according to the amount of income. (*Refer to current rates*) *Companies and other organisations* are liable for tax.

Queries about tax

Approach should be made to the appropriate tax office. Always quote your tax reference (this is written on documents from the tax office). Always keep copies of correspondence, including tax returns.

A number of explanatory leaflets are available from the tax office.

INDIRECT TAXATION

a) *VAT* (Value Added Tax) (*Refer Module 8*)
b) Other forms of indirect taxation include:
  (i) Customs and excise duties on tobacco and alcohol and on goods brought into the country.
  (ii) Road fund tax.
  (iii) Fuel tax on petrol or diesel oil.
c) Licences are required for a number of activities – television, driving, etc.

RATES

Rates are levied upon property – houses, flats, shops, factories and offices.
General rate: The money collected is used for public services – education, cleaning streets, library services, lighting, parks and gardens, etc.
Water, sewerage and environmental services have a separate rate.

Rateable value

This is decided by the local authority. If certain improvements are made to property, e.g. the addition of central heating or the building of an extension, rateable value is usually increased. An appeal about the assessment for rateable value may be made to the valuation officer of the local authority and a tribunal will decide if the assessment is to stand or if there can be a reduction.

General rate

The rate in the £ is fixed by the local authority. This amount multiplied by the rateable value of the property gives the amount to be paid as general rate for the year.
  Payment may be made in full, in two half-yearly instalments or by monthly instalments, according to arrangements with the local authority.

Water, sewerage and environmental services rate

The rate in the £ is fixed by the local water authority and this amount multiplied by the rateable value gives the rate to be paid for the year.

Payment may be made in full, in two or four instalments, or by saving 50p savings stamps. (Obtainable from the Post Office or council offices.)

Rate rebates

If the income of a household is below a certain sum, there may be entitlement to a rate rebate. Consult the finance department of the local authority or the social services.

Reduction in rates

Reduction may be made for facilities for a disabled person in the house.

NATIONAL INSURANCE

Contributions are made by employees and employers. (*Refer to p. 78*)

MONEY MANAGEMENT

Before there is a consideration of money management, certain terms need to be understood.

Inflation is a financial state in a country when the cost of goods and services overall are rising and there is less value for money. It is stated as a percentage rate.

Deflation is a financial state when the cost of goods and services are falling.

Retail Price Index (RPI) shows changes in the retail prices of goods and services by a comparison of average prices with those of a previous month. It is based on the needs of an 'average' family and can only provide a general guide to the cost of living.

Base Rate is the rate for short-term interest rates, e.g. bank rates and it influences all other interest rates, e.g. mortgage payments. The use of MLR (Minimum Lending Rate) ceased on 20th August 1981.

Interest is a sum of money paid when money or other assets are invested.

ASSETS

a) *Income*

  Family income or the income of an individual is the money from wages or salaries, interest from investment, and payments of various kinds which are received weekly or monthly or at other intervals. Income varies according to employment or unemployment, rises in salary or reduction in overtime, and changes in interest received. People who are self-employed may have great variations in income over a year.

b) *Capital*

Capital is money or assets owned by a person or a family. It may be money in a bank or in a building society, or invested in stocks and shares or kept at home. As well as money, there are other assets which can be considered as capital – a house, equipment and furnishings; a car; clothes, jewellery and antiques.

BUDGETING

Budgeting is the allocation of assets. In drawing up a budget, assets and expenditure need to be considered in relation to the style of living, e.g. the priorities for a young couple setting up a home will be different from a couple with one or more children.

Budgeting procedure

CONSIDERATION OF ASSETS

a) Income – wages/salary; child benefit; interest.
b) Capital in money – whether this is available or is tied up for a long or short term.
c) Accommodation – owned; on mortgage; rented.
d) Possessions – furniture; equipment; furnishings; clothes; car. Paid for or on credit.
e) Skills – to make articles or decorate the home.

CONSIDERATION OF AREAS OF EXPENDITURE

Essentials	*Decisions*
Rent or mortgage.	To buy or rent. Amount to pay.
Rates/ground rent.	Amount depends on decisions above.
Insurance – life, house structure (if owner), house contents, car (if owned).	How much insurance cover to take out.

Essentials	Decisions
Health – money for prescriptions, first aid box.	Private medical care.
Food – basics.	More expensive foods.
Heating – basic.	Extra heating.
Clothes – basics.	Non-essential/fashion clothes. To make or buy.
Household furniture, furnishings, equipment – basics.	To change frequently. To buy new or secondhand. To make home furnishings or buy ready-made.
Cleaning materials.	To try more expensive brands. To bulk-buy.
Home decoration – exterior, interior.	To change decoration frequently. Need for protection of structure. To do-it-yourself.
Home repairs – potentially dangerous/essential.	When it is safe to do-it-yourself or more economical than a professional repair.
Travel – work; school; shopping.	Car or public transport. Bicycle; Motorbike; Moped.
School expenses – meals, travel.	Private education.
Telephone.	Luxury or essential.
Licences – car; television; dog.	Necessities or non-essentials.
Garden – if available.	Bare maintenance. Expensive plants, etc. Food production. Children's play area.
Anniversaries. Special occasions – Christmas.	Limited or expensive provision.
Leisure activities necessary for health and relaxation.	Limited expenditure – parks; walking; libraries; radio or television, record player or tape recorder. More expensive pursuits – travel; eating out; sports equipment; video recorder. Children's toys.

Essentials	Decisions
Personal expenditure – adults' spending money, children's pocket money.	How much should be allowed.
Credit payments.	How much can be allocated.
Savings.	
Emergencies.	

PRIORITIES IN BUDGETING

Consult as many members of the family as possible. Children need to learn the necessity of money management early in life.

a) Work out how much of the family income is needed for essentials.
b) Decide how the payment for essentials should be made – in a lump sum; by instalments; by credit for which interest is paid.
c) Calculate the money left and allocate this according to wishes of family members – note the need for money for emergencies.

BALANCING A BUDGET

The comparison of expenditure against income will indicate if there is money left for further expenditure or savings. If there has been an emergency there may be a need to withdraw savings.

KEEPING RECORDS

A file should be kept of all relevant documents – accounts; income tax; pay slips; house purchase; insurance; bank statements; credit arrangements; cheque stubs; personal documents, e.g. birth certificates. Keep copies of business correspondence. Keep receipts and guarantees. Keep records of the settlement dates for accounts or arrange with the bank to pay standing orders/direct debits.

BANKING

Banking began when people deposited gold coins for safekeeping in places such as the vaults of goldsmiths. Depositors received receipts. When they wished to use the gold for payment for goods or services the receipts were presented. The people who were paid usually put the gold back into the vaults. It was gradually realised that it would be safer and easier just to transfer the receipts. These were the first bank notes and eventually resulted in a type of cheque. The accumulation of gold left with the goldsmiths made it possible for them to lend the surplus to merchants at a rate of interest, so beginning the lending services of banks.

Advantages of using a bank

Public banks provide a safe way to store money.
Problems of carrying large sums of money or keeping money at home are solved.
Easy payment of accounts is possible.
Interest is given on some deposits.
(*Bank Services – Refer to pp. 87–88*)
The Bank of England was founded in 1694 and is the central bank. It is responsible to the Government for the control of the monetary system and the issue of bank notes for England and Wales. The Royal Mint produces coins for the United Kingdom and for other countries.
Merchant Banks are concerned with company and international finance and not with general banking services.
Commercial Banks (Joint Stock Banks) include all the familiar banks except the Trustee Savings Banks and the Post Office Banks. They have a range of depositing and lending facilities and offer a variety of services for money management. (*Refer to leaflets published by banks for details of the accounts and services*)
Clearing Bank refers to the function of a bank to 'clear' a cheque from the account of the person issuing the cheque to the person receiving the cheque. Some of the large commercial banks are clearing banks.
Trustee Savings Banks. Facilities for customers used to be limited to basic savings but now a wide variety of bank services are available (*Refer to leaflets from the TSB*). Trustee Savings Banks are part of the National Savings Movement, together with the Post Office.
National Savings Bank is run by the Government through a post office. The first £70 of interest in the ordinary account is tax free. There are limited bank services but advantages in opening hours. No bank statements are issued.
National Giro Bank is a Government bank which offers a cheap and easy way of transferring money by single payment or by standing order/direct debit, and of obtaining money on demand. The Giro system of payment may be used by a person without a Giro account by payment of a small fee at the Post Office. Some Social Security benefits are paid by Giro cheques.

Co-operative Bank is part of the Co-operative Wholesale Society movement. There are banking facilities for saving, payment and withdrawal during shop hours.

Types of account

a) *Savings account/ordinary account*
   Money can be taken out on demand, according to the balance. A small rate of interest is usually paid. No cheque book is provided. A bank book is generally provided.

b) *Deposit account*
   This is intended for money which can be left to earn interest until it is needed. Seven days' notice, or more, is required for a withdrawal. A bank book is provided by some banks but no cheque book. A higher interest rate is paid than for a savings account.

c) *Current account*
   This is a cheque-book service. No interest is paid. A charge is made for the services provided but most banks cancel the charges if a certain amount of money is held in the account.

A cheque is an instruction in writing from the account holder(s) to the bank to pay out a sum of money. Cheques can only be issued up to a sum agreed with the bank. If the sum is exceeded, the cheque will be returned 'refer to drawer'. Cheques can be made out to 'self' or 'cash' so that the account holder can obtain cash. Leaflets can be obtained from banks showing how a cheque book should be used.

Cheque card is issued to responsible customers of a bank to identify the person issuing the cheque. The amount to which a cheque may be written is stated. The card must be signed by the owner and kept in a safe place. The loss must be reported immediately to the bank.

Credit Card, e.g. Access, Barclaycard (Visa) offers credit facilities. Presentation of the card enables the payment for goods or services without the use of cash or a cheque. A form or bill is signed by the credit-card owner and is kept while a copy is sent to the bank by the seller. A monthly bank statement lists all the transactions and the amount owed. If this is not paid in full, interest is charged. A credit limit is stated. The card must be signed and kept in a safe place. The loss must be reported immediately to a bank. The use of a credit card can result in over-spending. (*Refer Module 8*)

d) *Budget account*

This is not available at all banks. Large regular bills, e.g. rates, fuel bills, are listed by the customer and the total sum is divided into 12 monthly amounts. This amount is paid from the customer's current account into the budget account each month. The customer has to make out a cheque to pay each bill when it is due. A charge is made for the service.

Standing orders/direct debits – regular orders for payment for rates or a subscription or a television rental, etc., may be arranged through a current account. The customer fills in a form and the bank makes the payment with a deduction from the account. A charge is made for the service unless there is a favourable balance in the account.

Other bank services

Most commercial banks provide – loans and overdrafts; executive and trustee services; investment service and advice; taxation advice; insurance advice and service; foreign currency and credit facilities; storage for valuables; night safe facilities; cash dispenser (at some branches); personal and business advice. Information about services is obtainable on leaflets and at the banks.

Bank statements are sent out to customers at intervals. They list the withdrawals and deposits which have been made and the bank charges, and state the balance in the account.

Over-drawing an account means that credit by cheque or credit card has been used for more than the deposit at the bank. Cheques will be returned marked 'refer to drawer', i.e. the cheque 'bounces'. The bank will notify the customer.

Overdraft. In certain circumstances, agreement may be made by a bank manager for an overdraft but a high rate of interest is payable.

Opening a bank account

a) Collect leaflets from banks and study the accounts and services available.

b) Visit a bank which has a branch within a convenient distance of where you live or work.

c) State your circumstances and requirements and you will be given advice about the best form of saving/investment.

d) You will be required to give the name of a referee before you open an account – a person who knows you and has a professional occupation, e.g. a doctor, minister, teacher, etc.

e) You will have to provide a specimen signature.

f) When the reference has been cleared, the account can be opened with a deposit.

g) Most large banks offer a year's free banking for school leavers, i.e. no bank charges are made.

Information about bank accounts and services is stated on leaflets from banks. Further information may be obtained from: The Secretary, The Bank Information Service, 10 Lombard Street, London EC3V 9AT.

SAVINGS AND INVESTMENT

Savings and investment are both concerned with the lending of money to the Government, banks or industry, and receiving money for the loan. Money can also be lent to individuals but when large sums are involved, security must be considered. *Saving* usually refers to short- or medium-term deposits at banks, etc. *Investment* is used to indicate long-term deposits in stocks and shares and bonds, etc.

Considerations before saving or investing

a) Amount of money available.

b) Saving or investing in a time of inflation.

c) Circumstances, e.g. a young couple saving for a home.

d) Capital available for withdrawal quickly or long-term investment which takes time for withdrawal.

e) The best return for the loan, i.e. interest.

f) The best growth in capital to provide money for the future and a guard against inflation.

g) No income tax to pay, e.g. National Savings Certificates. Is income tax taken from the interest before payment to the investor, e.g. building society investment?

h) Saving through a building society could be an advantage if a mortgage is contemplated.

i) Security for the investment.

Short-term saving

Advantages – It is easy to deposit and withdraw money. Money is readily available. Practically no risk to capital.

Disadvantages – Interest is less than for longer term saving. There is little hedge against inflation.

a) Ordinary or current accounts at a bank.

b) Deposit or share accounts at a building society.

Medium-term saving

Advantages – Better rates of interest and hedge against inflation. A reliable way of saving for major items. Practically no risk to capital.

Disadvantages – Problems in immediate withdrawal for emergencies. Interest could be lost if money is withdrawn before the term of agreement.

a) DEPOSIT ACCOUNTS
At a bank. (*Refer to p. 87*)

b) NATIONAL SAVINGS
  1. Bank deposits (*Refer to pp. 87–88*)
  2. *National Savings Certificates* (Normal Issues). Rate of interest varies according to the time held. No income tax is payable.
  3. *Index-linked National Savings Certificates.* Similar to normal issue in conditions but index-linked against inflation. (*Refer to leaflets from the Post Office for current information.*)
  4. *Premium Savings Bonds.* These do not provide interest but are entered for weekly and monthly draws. There are top weekly prizes of £100,000 and prizes range down to £50. Winning numbers are selected by ERNIE (Electronic Random Number Indicator Equipment).
  5. *Save As You Earn* (SAYE). An arrangement is made to pay regular amounts each month at a post office, through a bank or as deductions from pay, for a stated period, usually 5 years. Savings are index-linked and free from income tax.

c) BUILDING SOCIETIES (*Refer Book 2 – The Home*)
Building societies provide loans for the purchase of property. To obtain money for lending, they borrow from investors and interest is paid according

to the length of time and the terms on which the money is borrowed. Income tax is deducted by the society at the basic rate except for SAYE where no tax is payable. Types of investment vary with different societies – check with information brochures.

1. *Deposit or share accounts.* Mainly for short-term saving but more interest is payable if there is a time restriction on withdrawal.
2. *Term share/option share.* Investment is for a fixed period, usually of 1 to 5 years. The longer the period, the higher the interest.
3. *Save As You Earn (Refer to p. 90)*

Long-Term Investment

Advantages – Interest can be higher than other types of saving. There could be an increase in capital.
Disadvantages – There may be difficulties in buying and selling some types of investment and there may be a charge for purchase and disposal. Money is not available on demand. There could be a risk of losing capital.

a) STOCKS AND SHARES (*Refer to the financial columns of newspapers*)
Stock is issued by the Government or by a company. It is usually stated in multiples of £100 but the purchase price varies according to estimated value on the Stock Exchange. The year of repayment is stated and interest is fixed and paid twice a year. Profit, if any, comes from a rise in the market price of the stock.
Shares are an investment in a company. A dividend is paid, usually twice a year, on the profit made by a company. If the profits are high, there is a good dividend paid, and the value of the shares should rise and could be sold for a higher price. However, if the profits are low, there is usually a reduction in dividend and probably a reduction in the value of the shares.
The Stock Exchange is in London (and other capital cities). Stockbrokers buy and sell stocks and shares from jobbers for the public or companies at a fee. There are trading floors in large cities.
Government Stock (Marketable Securities). Stock on the National Savings Stock Register may be purchased by the public through the Post Office. (*Refer to leaflet from any Post Office*)

b) UNIT TRUSTS

Lump sums or regular amounts may be placed in a unit trust. The money is invested by the managers of the trust and the interest gained is returned to investors or re-invested for them. The amount invested in a trust is divided into units. The value of the units vary according to the success of the investment and the value on the Stock Exchange.

c) LOCAL AUTHORITY BONDS

Bonds are issued by local authorities for a stated period(s) with different rates of interest.

d) PROPERTY

This is considered to be a safe investment but there may be problems involved in letting, evicting bad tenants, repairs, payment of rates, and Capital Gains Tax. It is not easy to realise money quickly.

e) ANTIQUES AND JEWELLERY

These can be a safe investment in time of inflation provided that there is knowledge, or expert advice is taken. Pleasure can be obtained from the use of the investment. However, the risk of theft is great and insurance cover is high. Selling may not be as easy as buying.

f) ASSURANCE

Sound forms of long-term investment can be undertaken. (*Refer to pp. 96–97*)

Note: For any form of saving or investment take advice from a reputable person – a bank manager, an accountant, etc.

INSURANCE AND ASSURANCE

Insurance is a payment towards a form of indemnity, i.e. compensation if something happens – if a house and contents are damaged by fire; if property is stolen; if a car is in an accident.
Assurance is a payment to produce a benefit of money in the future.

Definitions

Policy is the document setting out terms of the insurance/assurance con-tract.
Premium is the sum paid to the insurance company. The sum varies accord-ing to the insurance cover.

Benefit is the sum payable when a claim is made.
With-profits is an arrangement when a sum based on the profits of an
   insurance company is added to the sum to be paid.
Non-profit is when only the sum insured is paid.
Bonus is the form in which a company distributes its profits in a with-profits
   policy.

Compulsory insurance

Minimum Motor Insurance (Road Traffic Act cover)
A legal liability for all mechanically driven vehicles to cover claims against
the driver for death or injury to anyone including any passengers in the
driver's car. This cover does not include injury to the driver holding the
insurance or damage to property or to any cars involved. (*Refer to p. 94*)
National Insurance (*Refer to pp. 78, 98–99*)
Employer's Liability
Most employers are required to insure against injury or death at work for
the employees.

Semi-compulsory insurance

Mortgage Loan Insurance
A building society or any association lending money for the purchase of
property usually requires a life insurance policy to be taken out in case the
borrower dies before the loan is repaid.
Private Pension Scheme
Many employees are required to join a private pension scheme.

Voluntary insurance/assurance

The amount undertaken by an individual or a family depends upon the life
style and the degree of risk involved and cover required. Much will depend
upon what can be afforded and so priorities must be decided.

INSURANCE

Householder's insurance

a) *Building policy* covers the structure only – a house or flat plus adjacent
   buildings such as garage, stables, etc. Rented accommodation should be

insured for structure by the landlord. (Business premises need a different insurance cover.)

b) *Contents policy* covers the contents but not the structure.

c) *Building and contents* policy combines (a) and (b) above.

d) *Householder's policy* is a comprehensive policy for structure and contents which offers advantages such as index-linking to allow for inflation, personal liability, no deduction for wear and tear, etc.

e) *All risks policy* is for valuables which have to be listed for the insurance company to verify. Insurance cover can be expensive.

Cover for householder's insurance is against damage caused by most eventualities – fire; explosion; lightning; earthquake; storm; flood; accidental impact by road vehicle or aeroplane; damage; theft; vandalism, etc. On most policies there is a requirement that the first, e.g. £15 or a percentage of the claim should be paid by the insurer for certain eventualities, e.g. flood, in areas most likely to be affected.

Fire risk buildings, e.g. thatched-roofed buildings, need extra cover. Householder's insurance is not cheap but it is most important not to under-insure as the cost of replacement of house and contents is high. Index-linked policies are an advantage because the insurance cover is linked to inflation. Insurance companies will provide guidance.

Car insurance (Including all mechanically powered vehicles)

a) *Minimum cover policy* (Road Traffic Act cover) is the requirement by law. It only insures against death or injury to people – not the driver. It does not cover any damage or theft. The policy holder is liable.

It should be noted that a Third party policy (below) is usually the minimum cover accepted by insurance companies.

b) *Third party policy*
  'First party' is the insured person.
  'Second party' is the insurer, i.e. the insurance company.
  'Third party' is the person making the claim.
  This policy includes death or injury to people as in (a) above.
  There is also cover for damage to another person's car or property.
  The policy does not include damage to the policy-holder's car or theft, but cover can usually be extended to cover theft or fire for an extra fee.

c) *Comprehensive policy*
  Includes the above benefits plus:
  Loss or accidental damage to the policy-holder's car.

Death or injury to the policy holder and his/her family. (A scale of benefits will be listed on the policy.)

A proportion of medical expenses.

Compensation for theft of car, and for theft of contents up to a limited amount with exclusion clauses against loss of money and some valuables. (Extra cover could be obtained.)

A claim cannot be made for breakdowns, punctures, etc.

People using cars for purposes outside pleasure and normal business will need extra cover.

Sometimes there are exclusion clauses, e.g. against windscreen breakage.

CHOOSING A POLICY

This depends upon the type of vehicle, the area in which it is to be driven and the record of the driver.

NO-CLAIM BONUS

This is given to a person who has had claim-free motoring. This increases according to the number of years, usually up to 60 percent after 4 years. The bonus may be withdrawn in the case of an accident.

RAC OR AA MEMBERSHIP

This is a protective cover in case of a breakdown. For an extra fee, relay cover may be obtained. (*Refer to information from the Associations*)

TAKING A CAR ABROAD

Information must be obtained about the cover required. Check with the Insurance company.

CERTIFICATE OF INSURANCE

This must, by law, be up-to-date. It is required to be shown to the police, and used to obtain a Road Fund Licence.

Holiday insurance

This can cover cancellation, death or injury, medical expenses, loss or damage to luggage – except for valuables unless specified. There is a limit of payment according to premium. Cover could be limited to death or injury but it must be noted that medical costs are very expensive in some countries.

Accident or sickness insurance

This can be taken out in addition to the cover provided through the National Health Insurance. Policy arrangements depend upon the insurer's requirements. There are restrictions for the chronically sick, those in dangerous employment and the elderly.

Medical expenses insurance

This is taken out by people who wish to have private medical treatment for themselves and their families. There will still be liability for National Insurance contributions under the usual terms.

Miscellaneous insurance

Insurance against eventualities of various kinds, e.g. bad weather for an outdoor fête, can be taken out with the agreement of an Insurance company.

ASSURANCE

Assurance is concerned with the provision of financial security for the individual and the family. Benefit to the people concerned depends upon the terms of the policy. Cover/protection begins with the payment of the first premium.

Life assurance is provision for dependents following the death of the breadwinner. Some policies are simple and only provide for death before the policy matures. Other policies include investment profits.

Term assurance/insurance

An insurance against death during the term of the policy. If the insured person survives this term, nothing is paid out.

Whole life assurance

A fixed sum is paid out whenever the insured person dies. The policy can start at different age levels up to a fixed age. The amount of the premium depends upon the time the policy is to run and the sum to be paid out. Policies can be with-profits or non-profit.

Endowment assurance

Life assurance provides benefit for dependents. If the insured person wishes to derive benefit, an endowment policy should be taken out. This type of policy provides some insurance cover but it is mainly concerned with investment. If the insured person dies before the end of the term of the policy, the dependents receive a lump sum but if the insured person survives, the sum is still available to be collected. Various dates of maturity of policy can be chosen, e.g. the sum could be available for retirement, or the assurance may be linked to house purchase. Policies can be with-profits or non-profit.

Life assurance linked to unit trusts

Premiums paid are used for the purchase of unit trusts. If the insured person dies during the term of the policy, the units or a sum of money, or both, are paid to dependents. If the insured person survives, the units, or the value in cash, is paid out.

Annuity

In return for a sum of capital paid to a company, periodic payments are paid for the life of the assured, or for a fixed term. There are a number of variations in this type of policy.

Income tax relief

This is deducted at source by the insurance companies for policies over a certain value.

CHOOSING INSURANCE/ASSURANCE

a) Decide how much insurance is needed.
b) Try to work out how much assurance/investment is required.
c) Examine brochures from insurance companies.
d) Consult an insurance company with a branch near your home or work.
e) Note the insurance/assurance provided and consider the premiums.
f) A combined 'pack' may be available which includes various forms of cover at a reduced premium.

g) Do not enter into contracts for too much insurance when the premiums cannot be afforded.

h) Note the conditions of insurance policies – some people may not be accepted for certain policies; not telling the truth may result in claims not being paid.

Problems in paying premiums

Consult the insurance company immediately. The social services may be of assistance.

FINANCIAL PROVISION BY THE COMMUNITY

National Insurance provides certain benefits in return for regular contributions.

Class 1 contributions

People who work for an employer pay these contributions, as does the employer. For sufficient contributions the following benefits are available:
unemployment benefit; redundancy payments; sickness benefit; retirement pension; industrial injury benefit; industrial death benefit; death grant; widow's benefits; maternity benefit; guardian's allowance; child's special allowance. (Check current benefits.)

Class 2 contributions

The self-employed can pay these contributions.
Benefits as above are available except for:
Unemployment benefit; redundancy payments; industrial death benefit; child's special allowance.
Information about other classes of contributions and the benefits can be obtained from the Department of Health and Social Security.

BENEFITS

Earnings-related Supplement
This may be payable in addition to unemployment benefit, sickness benefit, maternity allowance and possibly industrial injury benefit, but only up to 85 per cent of reckonable weekly earnings. The supplement is paid for up to 6 months. (*Refer to leaflet NI 155A*)

Family Income Supplement
This is a payment for the employed, including the self-employed, if income is below a certain level. (*Refer to leaflet FIS 1*)
Unemployment benefit (*Refer to leaflet NI 12*)
Supplementary benefit
This may be claimed by people who do not have enough to live on and are:
  over pension age; unfit for work; unemployed and cannot get work; working only part-time; looking after a disabled relative; bringing up children alone. (Ask at a social security office.)
Social Security Benefits (*Refer to leaflet NI 196*)
Many benefits are available for people whether they are insured or not. Benefits include:
  National Health Service treatment; family planning; family income supplements; supplementary allowances; rent and rates rebates; industrial injury payments.
Other Benefits may be available
Free dental treatment, glasses, prescriptions. Free milk for young children and expectant mothers.

Claiming benefits

a) Go to the appropriate office – Unemployment Benefit Office; Job Centre; Social Security Office.
b) A Citizens Advice Bureau will help in case of doubt.
c) Take any appropriate documents, e.g. from a former employer.
d) Note any instructions about procedure.
e) Ask for advice if unsure. Collect explanatory leaflets.
f) Read any documents which you are required to sign or ask for them to be explained to you.
g) Note the dates of any appointments.
h) Inform the appropriate office about any change in circumstances.

Benefits for the Elderly
A number of benefits exist, e.g. travel facilities. Check with the local authority.

Voluntary Community Assistance
There are a number of voluntary agencies offering assistance especially for the elderly, e.g. Meals on Wheels. Check with the local voluntary associations.

MODULE SEVEN REFERENCES

Leaflets from the Tax Department.
Brochures from banks and the Post Office.
Brochures from building societies.
Brochures from insurance companies.
Leaflets from an Unemployment Benefit Office; a Social Security Office.

FOLLOW-UP ACTIVITIES

1. Investigate the services which are financed through rates and find out the percentage of rate which is used.
2. Work out a personal budget.
3. Collect brochures from banks. Examine the services which they offer.
4. Consider the type of saving which you might undertake.
5. Examine insurance policies. Note the cover which is stated, the premium, any exclusion clauses.

THE CONSUMER

HISTORY

A consumer is a user of goods and services for which cash has been taken or credit arranged. (Strictly speaking, a manufacturer is also a user of goods and services.)

Efforts to protect consumers against poor quality goods and services have been in evidence for centuries. The Romans placed lead seals on wine casks and legislated on food pricing; the Magna Carta laid down the first rules regarding the size of a loaf of bread; the mediaeval guilds took great care to ensure that their members did not produce and sell shoddy goods or offer substandard services to the public. Punishments for infringement of these laws or codes of practice were severe. The offender could be placed in the pillory or dragged through the streets with inferior merchandise hung around his neck or suffer the loss of an ear.

Up to the Victorian era there was little statutory protection for the consumer. The purchaser needed to inspect the goods thoroughly to be sure they were of sound quality. The phrase 'caveat emptor' (let the buyer beware) was the advice given to intending purchasers. Gradually, foundations were laid for the present statutory and voluntary regulations which protect the consumer today.

Post-war social and economic changes have provided the ideal climate for the growth of the consumer protection movement because:

a) After a period of war-time shortage and austerity, the income of consumers rose, enabling them to purchase many more products and services.

b) Consumers had a wider choice of goods and services.

c) New products were unfamiliar to consumers.

d) Some manufacturers did not provide information.
e) Retailers changed their patterns of selling, reducing personal service in their stores.

In 1957 The Consumers' Association was established. Consumers had access to information about products and services which formerly had been available only to manufacturers and retailers.

The growth of the consumer protection movement has meant:
a) Information available to the consumer about products and services has greatly improved.
b) Controls of trading practices have become stricter.
c) Legal rights of the consumer have improved.

CONSUMER PROTECTION AND LEGISLATION

The consumer is protected against poor quality merchandise by Acts of Parliament which prohibit inefficient service; hygiene below required standards; misleading advertising. The nature of consumer protection law is complex. The consumer should derive protection through both criminal law and civil law.

Criminal law is concerned with offences against the laws of the country. When a crime is committed (e.g. selling food on premises where hygiene is below the required standards) prosecution results. This may be by the police, or, if the consumer protection law is breached, by a trading standards officer. If criminal charges are proven the offender will be convicted and can be imprisoned or fined or both.

Civil law is concerned with disputes between private individuals and/or companies. If there is a breach of civil law (e.g. clothes damaged by a faulty washing machine) the individual can seek redress by suing the offender. This could result in damages or some other form of compensation.

DEVELOPMENT OF CONSUMER LAW

Although consumers have had some protection in law since ancient times there was little guarantee of standards, especially with weight and measurement, until the Weights and Measures Act 1878. There were only minor developments until 1952 when the Hodgson Committee investigated weights and measurement standards. Their recommendations resulted in the 1963 Weights and Measures Act; weights and measures departments were set up in each local authority, later renamed trading standards or consumer protection departments. Because of growing public concern about consumer protection, the Molony Committee was set up in 1959. Recommendations of the Committee are recognised as being the basis for current consumer protection rights.

Current consumer legislation is concerned with:

a) Safeguarding against deceptive and unfair trading practices.
b) Providing certain rights regarding the purchase and sale of goods and services with respect to: quality, quantity, performance, service, price information, credit facilities.
c) Setting out the duties and rights of consumers and merchandisers relating to: new technology, innovations in marketing, novel trading standards.
d) Stating health and safety standards.
e) Providing a means of redress if rights are infringed.
f) Making provision for information and advice on consumer matters to be readily available through organisations concerned with consumer protection.

Many Acts of Parliament make specific provision for the manufacture, distribution, description and sale of goods and services. Responsibility for seeing that this legislation is enforced is with the trading standards or consumer protection departments of local authorities.

SUMMARY OF MAJOR ACTS

Legislation	Main Elements

1893 Sale of Goods Act as amended to 1973 Supply of Goods (Implied Terms) Act and restated as 1977 Unfair Terms Act.	1. Merchandising of faulty goods and services.
	2. Seller must have right to sell.
	3. Goods must be
	  a) as described;
	  b) 'fit for purpose';
	  c) 'of merchantable quality'.
	4. Sellers have redress against suppliers/ manufacturers for defective goods.

Legislation	Main Elements
	5. Seller cannot exclude/limit liability for negligence which results in death/personal injury. 6. Onus on seller to prove 'exclusion' clauses are fair and reasonable. 7. Consumers' rights applicable whether transaction involves cash/credit/trading stamps.
1955 Food and Drugs Act.	1. Regulations concerning: quality, description, hygiene, labelling, composition. 2. Concerns health and safety of consumer.
1961 Consumer Protection Act (Molony Committee) as amended *1971 Consumer Protection Act.*	1. Concerns health and safety of consumer. 2. Empowers Secretary of State for Prices and Consumer Protection to make regulations regarding product safety standards on: composition, construction, design, labelling. 3. Redress from manufacturer and/or retailer.
1963 Weights and Measures Act (Hodgson Committee).	1. Quantity/weight must be indicated on many goods (e.g. food). 2. Certain goods must be sold in prescribed quantities. 3. Metrication to be gradually introduced. 4. Concerns health and safety of consumer.
1968 Trade Descriptions Act. *1972 Trade Descriptions Act* (replaced 1887–1953 *Merchandise Marks Acts*).	1. Prohibits false/misleading descriptions/ unauthorised claims of goods and services. 2. Goods (not medicines, dyes, etc.) made outside UK must indicate country of origin.
1971 Unsolicited Goods and Services Act. *1975 Unsolicited Goods and Services Act.*	1. Traders cannot demand payment for unordered goods. 2. Since 1975 Secretary of State may make regulations about wording and layout of agreements.

Legislation	Main Elements
1973 Fair Trading Act.	1. Protects against harmful trading practices.
	2. Secretary of State for Prices and Consumer Protection can make statutory orders.
	3. Set up a Consumer Protection Advisory Committee.
	4. Established post of Director General of Fair Trading.
	5. Made information and advice available through Office of Fair Trading.
	6. Encourages setting up of Codes of Practice by associations of traders for member companies.
1974 Prices Act. *1975 Prices Act.*	1. Unit pricing.
	2. Pricing policies on subsidised foods.
	3. Regulation of prices for food and household necessities.
	4. Price display regulations.
	5. Prevent/restrict increases in prices/charges.
1974 Consumer Credit Act (Crowther Committee).	1. Replaced earlier legislation on credit.
	2. Most radical reform of consumer credit law in United Kingdom.
	3. Controls dealings of all persons concerned with credit activities; cannot operate unlicenced – licences must be renewed every 3 years.
	4. 'Truth in lending' is main principle.
	5. Regulations made by Secretary of State for Prices and Consumer Protection.
	6. Director General of Fair Trading administers Act.
	7. Consumer is entitled to address of credit reference agency if refused credit.
1978 Consumer Safety Act.	1. Concerned with health and safety of consumer.
	2. Regulations classified: to protect children; to protect against poisons; to cover safety on heating and electrical goods.
	3. Supplier may be sued or prosecuted if goods bought cause injury/damage.

It is obvious that there are rapid changes in consumer protection and legislation, therefore it is essential for consumers, traders, suppliers and manufacturers to keep up to date.

CODES OF PRACTICE

These are voluntary codes whose purpose is to improve the standards of service of traders to consumers, but the codes do not offer any extra legal rights to consumers. The following are examples of some of the trading associations who have established voluntary codes of practice:

Asssociation of British Travel Agents.
Association of Manufacturers of Domestic Electrical Appliances.
Association of British Launderers and Cleaners.
National Association of Shoe Repair Factories.
Mail Order Traders' Association.
National Association of Retail Furnishers.

SELECTED INFORMATION AND ADVICE SERVICES

The Government, local authorities and the independent agencies dealing with consumer protection policy play a vital role in advising and helping consumers. Legislation is the responsibility of the Government, enforcement is the duty of local authorities.

The following organisations are concerned with consumer legislation and protection:

1. *Office of Fair Trading* (OFT) was set up by the 1973 Fair Trading Act, under the control of the Director General of Fair Trading. Some of the functions of OFT are:

a) to inform and educate consumers and produce a wide range of free publications;
b) to investigate unfair trading practices;
c) to institute legal proceedings against traders who contravene the law;
d) to act as an arbiter between consumers, traders and manufacturers.

2. *National Consumer Council* (NCC) is an independent organisation established in 1975. Members are appointed by the Secretary of State for Prices and Consumer Protection. The NCC:

a) represents views of all consumers to international, national and local bodies concerned with consumer protection;

b) acts as a consultant on consumer affairs;

c) does not deal with individual consumer complaints.

3. *Department of Prices and Consumer Protection* is headed by the Secretary of State for Prices and Consumer Protection. Its responsibilities include:

a) consumer protection and safety legislation;

b) establishing consumer advice centres;

c) publishing monthly (via the Information Division) a Consumer Information Bulletin for circulation to news media and other consumer organisations.

4. *Ministry of Agriculture, Fisheries and Food* is responsible for:

a) jurisdiction (law administration) concerned with food (advertising, labelling, composition);

b) public health standards for the milk and meat industries.

5. *Department of Health and Social Security* liaises with local authorities to promote and enforce hygiene and safety legislation, including medicines.

6. *The Home Office* is concerned with the safety of the consumer.

7. *Consumer Advice Centres* (CAC). The 1972 Local Government Act promoted local authorities to set up a network of Consumer Advice Centres. The 1973 Local Government Act gave Weights and Measures (Trading Standards) Authorities permission to offer consumer advice. The CAC:

a) give advice on consumer problems;

b) distribute free leaflets produced by OFT;

c) deal with complaints;

d) offer a lecture service;

e) give advice and help to retailers;

f) operate a mobile service in rural areas;

g) liaise with citizens' advice bureaux;

h) perform the advisory service of trading standards/consumer protection departments;

i) provide an out-of-hours consumer advice answering service in some areas.

8. *Trading Standards/Consumer Protection Departments* (originally weights and measures departments)

a) enforce consumer protection legislation;

b) counsel traders and manufacturers on their rights and responsibilities;

c) promote consumer information and education through consumer advice centres.

9. *Citizens' Advice Bureaux* were originally set up in 1939 to give advice

to the general public on war-time problems. Financed by a grant from the local authority. The service of free, independent and confidential advice includes:

a) a solicitor rota scheme (with agreement of Law Society);
b) dealing with health, housing, personal, social, legal and consumer problems and inquiries.

10. *Consumer/Consultative Councils in Nationalised Industries* include: energy (coal, solid fuel, electricity, gas), transport (air, road, rail, water) and the Post Office. They act as 'watchdogs' on behalf of the consumers. Addresses of gas and electricity councils are on the back of fuel bills. (*Refer Book 2 – The Home*)

11. *Consumer's Association* was established in 1957 to give impartial advice on goods and services. The organisation:

a) tests products;
b) investigates services;
c) publishes reports on products and services investigated;
d) produces:

Which?	Motoring Which?
Handyman Which?	Good Food Guide
Holiday Which?	Consumer education kits
Money Which?	Series of informative books;

e) reports to government departments and suppliers;
f) acts as consultant to Department of Prices and Consumer Protection;
g) is a member of the European Office of Consumers' Unions and of the International Organisation of Consumers' Unions.

12. *British Standards Institution* (*BSI*) (originally the Engineering Standards Committee) It:

a) sets up standards of quality and measurement and issues standards to manufacturers;
b) promotes international standards of quality and measurement;
c) co-ordinates efforts of consumers and manufacturers to improve standards;
d) produces information for school use.

Each British Standard test (there are over 7,000) indicates: dimension, performance, method of test, safety, terminology, codes of good practice.

The Kite mark is issued when goods conform to the standards laid down.
The Safety Mark is issued when goods conform to safety standards.
Manufacturers wishing to display these symbols on their goods must first

submit them to BSI for their rigorous test procedures and agree to have them re-tested and inspected regularly without warning.

13. *Design Council* – set up in 1944 under another name to try to ensure that the design of consumer goods was pleasing and that the goods were 'fit for their purpose'. In 1972 it was renamed The Design Council. There are permanent exhibitions in some large cities. A Design Index of goods is produced according to design, safety and performance. Manufacturers whose goods are listed can display the 'design label' on their products.

International Organisations are concerned with consumer advice, protection and representation; two are:

a) International Organisation of Consumer Unions (IOCU).

b) European Office of Consumers Unions.

THE DISTRIBUTION OF CONSUMER GOODS

The following diagram shows the paths of distribution for consumer goods.

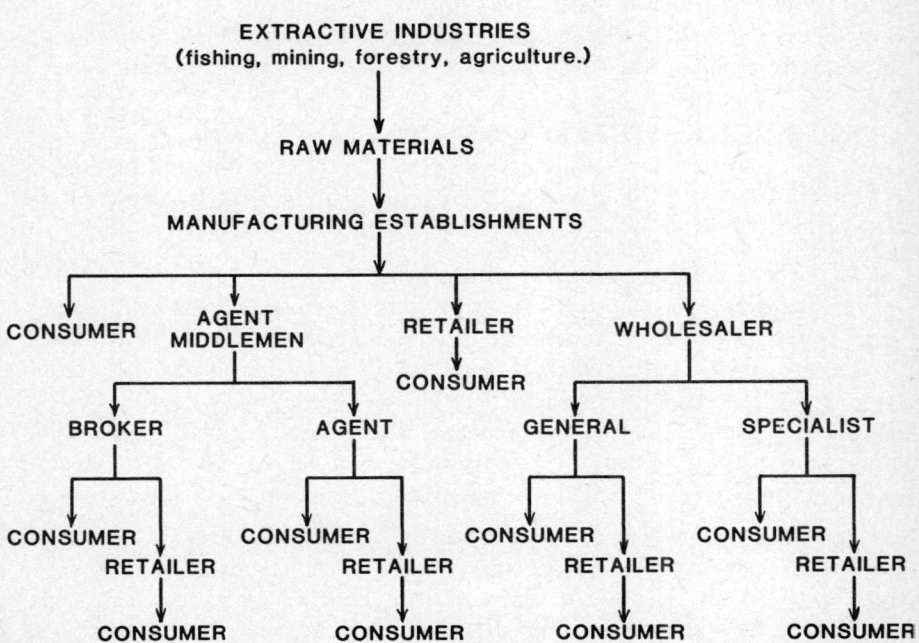

A *wholesaler* distributes goods. Functions may also include warehousing (a wide range of goods or a specialist section) financing, packaging, stabilising price levels, bulk order breaking.

An *agent middleman* may work for several manufacturers – Broker or one manufacturer – Agent. Both earn commission.

A *retailer* is the final link in the chain of production and distribution of goods and services. The table on p.p. 111 to 115 indicates the wide selection of retailers.

SHOPPING

Good shopping practice begins at home. Before going to the shops decide what is needed, consider how much money is available, check sizes and measurements, identify possible suppliers.

At the chosen suppliers check price and Value Added Tax.

There is a need also to check: method of payment, delivery, after-sales service or guarantee, facilities for exchange.

Purchasing goods and services is a compromise between: what is wanted, what money is available, what the supplier has available.

It is necessary to assess the goods and services available so that value for money and efficient service in pleasant surroundings can be obtained.

VALUE ADDED TAX (VAT)

VAT is a tax on spending. Some goods or services are:
a) Exempt, e.g. insurance.
b) Zero rated, e.g. food and books.
c) Rated at a percentage of the selling price.
Where payable, the tax is added at each successive stage of a transaction, e.g. from supplier to manufacturer to wholesaler to retailer to consumer.

Some businesses are *exempted* from the VAT scheme because their sales turnover is less than the prescribed level, but they must pay VAT on goods or services bought in for the business. A business required to pay VAT must be registered with the Customs and Excise Department for collection. A portion of the VAT paid by a registered business may be claimed back.

Type	Characteristics	Location	Examples of types of merchandise	Method of selling	Advantages	Disadvantages
A. STORE RETAILING 1. Market.	Oldest type of retail outlet; colourful.	Market place, in centre of towns and cities; in some shopping centres.	Food, clothing, shoes, accessories, flowers, animals, jewellery, hard-ware, antiques.	Personal service.	Possibly low cost of merchandise; great variety, flexible, possibly outdoors.	Can be difficult to follow up complaints; quality variable, may be weekly; bad weather.
2. Speciality store.	a) One type of product/service; possibly shopkeeper is owner. b) Fuel showrooms.	High street of village, town, city; shopping centre or precinct.	a) confectionery, greengroceries, fish, flowers, groceries, clothes, shoes, sweets, chemist, jewellery, household goods, hairdresser, books. b) Gas/electricity/solid fuel appliances.	Personal service.	Personal relationships with clientele; longer opening hours. Range of goods/advice for stated fuel.	Can be expensive; small selection of merchandise; can lack modern facilities. Goods displayed are not always for sale.
3. Chain store.	More than 10 branches of speciality shops; strong corporate identity.	High street; shopping precinct.	Confectionery, food, clothing, shoes, household goods, books, drinks.	Self-service.	Variety of goods in one store; relatively low prices; own brands; good customer relationship policy; no pressure to buy; goods readily exchanged if faulty.	Few extra services; location of goods takes time; centralised check-out, can take long time; can be tempted to make impulse purchases.

Type	Characteristics	Location	Examples of types of merchandise	Method of selling	Advantages	Disadvantages
4. Department store.	Sell four or more different types of consumer goods in separate departments, usually in one building; female clothing is generally one of the departments	High street of larger towns and cities; shopping centre.	Clothing, household goods, cosmetics, shoes, food, haberdashery, furniture, hair/beauty salon, travel agents.	Self and personal service.	Usually little pressure to buy; offer extra services, e.g. free delivery in certain areas; credit facilities; cloakrooms; restaurants; coffee shops; making up soft furnishings; staff expertise on various types of merchandise.	Prices can be high; cost of travel.
5. Co-operative Society store	Owned by customers; dividends paid to customers on money spent – this can be drawn or saved with interest accruing.	Village, town, city, high street shopping precinct/centre; mobile delivery service.	Food, clothing, footwear, furniture, household goods, drinks, chemist, travel agent, milk, bread, coal, hairdressing.	Self, and personal service.	Supplied by own wholesale society; own brands; service facilities; restaurant/ coffee shop, dividends; organise social activities for members; bank during shopping hours.	Small societies can lack modern facilities.

6. Discount store.	Cut-price goods, may be in specially built premises or in converted warehouses.	Usually outskirts of towns and cities.	Food, household equipment, furniture, audio/visual equipment.	Self-service.	Low prices; some goods are own brands; good car parking; may have cut-price petrol. Some have restaurants; can buy in bulk.	Own transport usually necessary. Can be for 'trade' customers only.
7. Hyper-market.	Very large supermarket.	Outskirts of towns; cities.	Food, household goods, clothing, drinks.	Self-service.	Good car parking; low prices; merchandise under one roof.	Travel problems.
8. Take-away food shop.	Food cooked ready to eat; usually foreign foods.	High street of towns, cities.	Food.	Personal service.	Open late hours; convenient for people who lack interest, facilities or time for cooking.	Can be expensive; danger in time between purchasing and eating, particularly if reheated.
9. Mobile van.	Usually owner-driven.	Covers a particular area; can have an established list of customers.	Green-groceries, food, toiletries, household cleaning materials.	Personal service.	Convenient for shoppers who cannot travel to shops.	Can be expensive, small selection.

B. NON-STORE RETAILING

Type	Characteristics	Location	Examples of types of merchandise	Method of selling	Advantages	Disadvantages
1. Mail order a) department store; b) chain store; c) direct mailing; d) agency; e) media.	Goods ordered by mail from catalogue/brochure/leaflet/newspaper/magazine.	Own home or home of agent.	Clothing, household goods, certain food products, toys, furniture, audio/visual equipment.	Agent or consumer response to catalogue or advertisement.	Can have use of goods before credit debt settled. Free delivery, goods on approval; arm-chair shopping.	Goods cannot be obtained immediately; no discount for cash; nuisance to return if wrong size; not always true to description; can be expensive.
2. Automatic vending.	Money put in machine displaying goods.	High street, leisure centres, airports, railway stations.	Drinks, cigarettes, chocolate, food, tights, sanitary protection.	Consumer.	No closing times.	Limited choice; can be expensive; needs to be maintained regularly.
3. 'Party'-merchandising.	Demonstration held in private home or at private function with refreshments.	Usually in private home.	Plastic containers, jewellery, clothing, stainless steel.	Agency and commission usually in form of merchandise being demonstrated is given to party organiser.	Can be held in evenings, social gatherings; can be less expensive than in store.	May feel obligation to purchase merchandise or give a 'party'; may be problems in exchanging goods; can be delay in obtaining goods ordered from central warehouse; may be expensive.

| 4. Door-to-door selling. | Travelling salesman. | Can have a 'round' of established customers, or new area. | Encyclopaedias, brushes, cosmetics, household cleaners, milk, bread, double glazing. | Personal service. | May be regular contract, goods delivered to door. | Can feel obligation to purchase; some salesmen are very persistent and use persuasive techniques; can be expensive; may be problems in exchanging goods and after-sales service. |

CONTRACTS

Throughout life, agreements are made which are legally enforceable. These agreements are called *contracts*. People are usually aware that a contract is made in the case of house purchase but the purchase of a magazine, a bus ride or a loaf of bread all constitute the making of a contract between a buyer and a seller.

A *verbal contract* is sufficient to be legally enforceable for some contracts.

A *written agreement* is the law for other contracts (e.g. house purchase).

Silence may constitute a contract (e.g. purchasing goods from an automatic vending machine).

In legal terms there are seven essentials in a contract.

Essentials of a legal Contract	Explanation
1. 'Offer'.	An offer is usually made by the purchaser.
2. 'Acceptance'.	An acceptance is usually made by the seller.
3. 'Consideration'.	There is a promise to pay for the goods or services.
4. 'The intention to create legal relations'.	A binding agreement which results in legal action if there is failure to keep it.
5. 'Parties must have the capacity to contract'.	Most adults can make contracts but there are restrictions on several categories of people: those below legal age and those without legal responsibility, e.g. mentally ill.
6. 'The contract must be legal and possible'.	A contract is not legal or possible if it is: a) illegal; b) immoral; c) contrary to public policy.
7. 'Both parties must genuinely consent to the terms of the contract'.	There must be no error, no fraud, no misrepresentation, no duress and no undue influence by either party.

HIRING OF GOODS

The following relates to whether goods or equipment are hired on a short-
or long-term basis. Clothing, do-it-yourself household equipment, books
and audio–visual equipment are covered by the contract agreed by the
consumer and hirer. The contract may be verbal or written.

A verbal agreement means that the consumer must take 'reasonable' care of
the goods/equipment. The terms will vary according to the type of agreement.

A written agreement cannot be enforced unless it is in the prescribed manner
set out in the Consumer Credit Act 1974. Section 101 of this Act enables
the hire agreement to be terminated after 18 months. However, it is most
important that the agreement is studied carefully *before* signing to make
sure the terms of the agreement are 'reasonable'.

PURCHASING SERVICES

When a service is bought it is a skill that is purchased. Hairdressing, building, decorating, dry cleaning, shoe repairing, car repairing/maintenance,
using a travel agent to book a holiday, are all services. The contract made
depends on the terms stated and agreed between the buyer and the seller. It
is important to state exactly what work is to be done in writing at the outset,
since the consumer does not have to pay for work which is unauthorised.

'CAVEATS' FOR THE CONSUMER

The majority of services performed are carried out to the satisfaction of
both parties to the contract, however, note the following:

1. **Price**
a) *estimate* – guide to the cost; final price may be different to estimate.
b) *quotation* – fixed price, binding on both parties.
c) *paying in advance* – never pay whole amount until the work is complete
   and satisfactory; do not pay more than a 'reasonable' amount in advance.
d) *call-out charge.* – does not include the cost of the work; it is payment for
   inspection and estimate.
2. **Time**
a) *limit* – should be stated. If service is not performed by the date set,
   claim redress/compensation or refuse to pay until completion.

b) *broken appointments* – if the workmen fail to keep appointment, the consumer can claim redress.
3. **Standard of work**
   – the standard of work must be 'reasonable'; materials must be suitable; if not, claim redress.
4. **Liability**
a) for death/personal injury as a result of negligence on part of supplier of service cannot be restricted or excluded.
b) for loss/damage to property as a result of negligence on part of supplier of service can be excluded if exclusion clause deemed 'reasonable'.
5. **Alterations**
   which are considered 'reasonable' can be made.

SALE GOODS AND OFFERS

Consumers are protected by the 1968 Trade Descriptions Act and Sale of Goods Act 1893 [as amended Supply of Goods (Implied Terms) Act 1973].
a) Price reduction must be genuine, i.e. the original higher price must have been displayed continuously for a period of 28 days within the previous 6 months.
b) Goods which have been bought in specially for the sales period must not give an impression of being price reduction goods.
c) Seller must not claim the price to be lower than the manufacturer's recommended price unless it is true.
d) Sales goods must be of 'merchantable quality' unless defects are indicated.
Note: It is inadvisable to order goods by mail from some firms which offer a large price reduction. If the goods are ordered through a *free* leaflet, the Mail Order Protection Law may not be enforceable.

ADVERTISING

Advertising is one of the greatest influences concerned with choice of goods and services. As well as the legal regulations on advertising, the British Code of Advertising Practice is a source of voluntary control. It is administered by the Advertising Standards Authority and comprises people from the media, business management and independent individuals who are connected with advertising currently, or have been so in the past. When an individual believes the code to be breached, a complaint, with a copy of the offending advertisement, may be sent to the Advertising Standards

Authority. They can require the advertisement to be amended or withdrawn if they consider the code to be contravened.

The objectives of advertising are:

a) To make the product known through visual, literal or oral means, or a combination;
b) To persuade the consumer to buy a product or service or to make the consumer develop or change a habit;
c) To create an image of a company or a political party.

The techniques used by an advertiser to fulfil the objectives are carefully selected for the potential market. They may include the use of: fashion; famous people; easily identifiable jingles or characters; humour; children; animals; family life; young love; prestige in work or 'keeping up with neighbours'; scientific image.

Groups who receive advertising

a) Potential buyers – consumers with a strong likelihood of making a purchase because they have the necessary resources.
b) Future buyers – consumers who cannot buy now because they have no resources or they are too young.
c) Actual buyers/owners – this group is most observant about the advertising claims for goods.
d) Persons who influence groups of buyers – these may be: parents; close relatives; friends; social class groups; teachers; other professionals; retailers.
e) Distributors and suppliers – these include traders; sales representatives.
f) Employees of manufacturers/service industries: some companies produce advertising literature specially designed for their employees.

Advertisements are placed:

a) On television.
b) On radio.
c) In newspapers, magazines and trade journals.
d) On hoardings (street, railway stations).
e) In educational material produced by companies/organisations.
f) On public transport, in shop windows, on parking meters.
g) In leaflets or brochures.

It must be obvious that the cost of advertising adds to the price of goods and services. It is important that consumers consider advertisements carefully and are not persuaded by the image presented in an advertisement to purchase goods and services which they do not really want or are not suited to their purpose.

METHODS OF CREDIT

There are two ways a consumer can obtain credit:
a) Borrow a sum of money and pay it back later.
b) Order goods or services and pay later or over a period of time.
Currently the 1974 Consumer Credit Act covers all credit transactions up to £5,000. All interest and credit charges must be calculated by a standard method to help the consumer to compare the cost of borrowing. All credit dealers must state:
a) APR (annual percentage rate of the total charge for credit) in advertisements, quotations, price tags.
b) Total cost of loan.
c) Cash price.
The following regulations apply to all written credit agreements:
a) Size and style of lettering.
b) Colour of paper.
c) Number of hand-written words.
d) Borrower must be able to read whole agreement before signing.
e) Rights and duties of borrower and lender.
f) Total cost of loan and APR.
g) Redress if dissatisfaction.
h) Cancellation date.
i) Terms of transaction.
j) Borrower must be given signed copy and a copy signed by lender within 7 days.
k) Agreement legal from date of posting by lender.
l) Borrower cannot be sued until agreement in possession.
m) All agreements can be cancelled, withdrawn from, or terminated and special conditions apply to each.
It is unlawful for women who are in employment to be discriminated against when seeking credit. A woman who is not working and seeking credit must receive the same treatment as an unemployed man seeking credit, i.e. a

guarantor must be named. A guarantor undertakes to honour the debts/ promises of a debtor. THE LIABILITY SHOULD BE NOTED.

Basically there are two types of credit:

1. *Purchaser credit* – a borrower purchases goods/services from a lender or from a supplier who has a business arrangement with the lender. If the goods are faulty, the supplier *and* the lender can be sued. The contract is a 'debtor–creditor–supplier' agreement.

2. *Loan credit* – a borrower receives a loan of money. The lender cannot be sued if goods bought with the loan are faulty. The contract is a 'debtor–creditor' agreement.

Credit options	*Conditions*

1. *Bank Loan*
    a) overdraft;
    b) ordinary loan;
    c) personal loan;
    d) budget account.
	Can overdraw money to a set limit from current account. Interest rates vary;
	Interest rates vary;
	Interest rate fixed for loan period;
	    (i) annual household bills totalled;
	    (ii) bills paid by standing order;
	    (iii) repayments spread over year;
	    (iv) service charge can be high.

2. *Credit cards*
    a) Bank (e.g. Barclay card. Access card).
	May be:
	    (i) used to endorse cheque and no interest payable;
	    (ii) obtained from own bank;
	    (iii) used for cash/goods/services;
	    (iv) used abroad;
	    (v) individual credit limit.
	            (*Refer Module 7*)

b) Store budget/subscription/ revolving account.	(i) customer agrees monthly repayment amount
	    (ii) amount which can be spent at store is multiple of monthly amount according to store's arrangement, e.g. monthly repayment £20, ceiling credit amount £200, once ceiling credit of £200 reached, 2 months repayment could allow further credit of £40;
	    (iii) monthly statement includes interest;

option.	(i) can settle monthly debt and pay no interest; (ii) can repay minimum amount monthly and pay interest.

Credit options	Conditions
3. *Credit Sale.*	a) written agreement if more than £30; b) goods are property of borrower from date of purchase/date Agreement posted if over £30; c) seller cannot repossess if instalments not paid; d) seller can sue for debt owed; e) APR can be high.
4. *Credit union.*	a) groups with common bond, e.g. place of work; b) for saving/seasonal/emergency loan; c) non-profit making.
5. *Finance company personal loan.*	a) minimum loan £100 or £200; b) APR often quite high; c) terms vary; d) usually some security required. CONSIDER CAREFULLY FINANCIAL IMPLICATIONS OF SUCH A LOAN. SEEK ADVICE BEFORE ENTERING INTO CONTRACT.
6. *Hire purchase.*	a) may be with supplier; b) may be with finance company; c) goods hired until last instalment paid; d) goods can be repossessed; e) goods cannot be sold until debt is paid; f) APR can be high; g) written agreement; h) pay deposit and weekly/monthly instalments.
7. *Insurance policy loan.*	a) given on endowment/whole life policies; b) loan up to 90 per cent of current cash-in value of policy; c) can repay when policy due if continue to pay monthly premiums and pay annual interest; d) can repay on maturity date, but more expensive.

Credit options	Conditions
8. *Mail order catalogue.*	a) take delivery of goods and repay, usually weekly, over 20 or 38 weeks; b) larger items can have HP agreements; c) no discount for cash.
9. *Moneylender.*	a) may or may not want security for loan; b) interest rates usually very high; c) repayments generally weekly. CONSIDER CAREFULLY FINANCIAL IMPLICATIONS OF SUCH A LOAN. SEEK ADVICE BEFORE ENTERING INTO CONTRACT. ENSURE LENDER HAS LICENCE.
10. *Trading cheques/ vouchers.*	a) usually for clothing; b) working agreement between trading company and local shops; c) agent gives voucher for up to £30; d) debt repaid weekly over 20 weeks or longer; e) interest charge quite high; f) service charge.

LABELLING

The Molony Report in 1959 recommended that labelling should be compulsory. Some progress with laws and regulations has been made but for the most part labelling remains a voluntary decision by manufacturers and traders. The European Economic Community is developing a policy on labelling for all member states.

The *consumer* requires labels: to help in choice (e.g. price, country of origin); to provide information about installation and use, safety precautions, care routines/maintenance.

The *trader* requires labels: to identify goods, to enable repeat orders, to aid shop assistants to provide information for the buyer, to aid security and help prevent theft.

The information on labels found on goods manufactured or sold in the United Kingdom can be classified:

a) *Facts* may include
  (i) price/unit price on food/VAT.
  (ii) dimensions (width/length/height/depth/capacity/dress size).
  (iii) ingredients with generic names and additives (food/drugs/cosmetics/ content of fibre/fabric finish).
  (iv) date ('sell-by'/'best use before').
  (v) energy consumption (electrical appliances).
  (vi) country of origin.
b) *Care instructions* may include procedure for: washing, drying, dry cleaning, ironing/pressing, maintenance. (*Refer* Book 2 – The Home)
c) *Performance details* indicate the ability of the product to carry out stipulated tasks.
d) *Safety details* warn against hazards and indicate correct procedure for use. Regulations are being prepared so that safety labels will be design and colour coded according to: prohibition, mandate, conditions of safety.
e) *Theft prevention* Some stores attach a special label which can only be removed with a special instrument at the payment desk. If labels are not removed (e.g. during shoplifting) then electronic beam on store exit is broken and staff alerted to the theft.
   Labels may be stuck on, firmly attached, swing ticket, woven into the fabric.
f) *Barcode*
   This is a 13-digit code included on the labels of a wide variety of goods. The code is scanned at the check-out desk so a record of the sale is made which is then available for:
  (i) the trader – for accounting, restocking, reordering.
  (ii) the consumer – for an itemised record of purchases; to monitor price changes; for a future shopping list.

Further developments in computer labelling will enable products to be easily identified. There may be a link with computer selling.

GUARANTEES

A guarantee is a voluntary promise by the supplier/manufacturer to repair or replace a defective product if the fault occurs within a stated period. It is given in addition to the rights under the 1893 Sale of Goods Act. The terms of the guarantee are varied and it is necessary to read individual guarantees to be sure what is promised. In law, guarantees do not have to be signed and returned to the manufacturer, but it is advisable. A guarantee may aid a claim from the manufacturer for redress for supplying faulty goods if:

a) the goods were a gift;
b) the seller is not traceable;
c) the seller has ceased trading.

Seek advice from one of the consumer protection agencies if in doubt about making a claim under guarantee for faulty goods.

COMPLAINTS PROCEDURE

Making a complaint can be less difficult if the consumer is aware of his legal rights and follows the procedure outlined.

Goods

1. All goods sold must be:
   a) of merchantable quality;
   b) as described;
   c) 'fit for purpose'.
2. A contract of sale is usually between the consumer and the trader.
3. When goods are faulty the consumer may:
   a) receive a cash refund;
   b) receive a replacement;
   c) have a repair done free of charge;
   d) obtain a cash payment for the difference between the cash paid and the value of the faulty goods.
4. A consumer has no redress if:
   a) faults were indicated at time of purchase;
   b) goods were examined and faults noticed at time of purchase;
   c) there is a change of mind about the purchase;
   d) damage is deliberate;
   e) the goods were received as a present – the claim must be made by the actual purchaser.

Services

1. All services performed must be carried out carefully and in a 'workmanlike manner'.

2. If damage or injury results, or incorrect procedure is adopted, then there is a right to compensation.

3. A contract should indicate a time factor for completion.

For both goods and services there is a legal time limit in which to claim redress.

Outline procedure:

1) Always retain receipts/contracts – they are usually required to obtain redress.
2) Stop using goods as soon as fault appears.
3) List points of complaint to be made (e.g. date of purchase, faults).
4) Inform the trader calmly as soon as possible:
a) in person – ask for the manager/owner and take the receipt or proof of purchase and take portable goods – DO NOT HAND OVER GOODS WITHOUT A RECEIPT;
b) by telephone – note date and time of call and name of person taking the call;
c) by letter enclosing a copy or details of receipt – keep the original receipt safely.
5) If no satisfaction, ask to see/speak to/write to someone in a senior position.
6) Note reason for refusal of redress and the name and position of person involved.
7) Consult (as appropriate)
a) trading standards/consumer protection department;
b) citizens advice bureau;
c) consumer/consultative council of national industry (if public services);
d) environmental health department (if food);
e) local consumer group;
f) solicitor.
g) Take complaint to small claims court after seeking advice from a knowledgeable person.

WARNING – the complaint must be reasonable and genuine because there will be limited chance of redress if a garment that is too small, splits on wearing or if boots which are sold as 'not waterproof' let in water on wearing in stormy weather.

THE EFFECT OF THE EUROPEAN ECONOMIC COMMUNITY ON THE CONSUMER

The UK joined the European Economic Community on 1st January 1973. The EEC aims to look at consumer protection policies and laws in all member states and make them applicable to every member. In April 1975 a programme was adopted by the Council of Ministers. It set out the basic rights of community consumers regarding:
a) health and safety;
b) protection of economic interests;
c) redress;
d) information and education in consumer matters;
e) representation.

EEC organisations affecting consumer affairs
Council of Ministers, European Commission, European Parliament, European Court of Justice, Consumers' Consultative Committee.

MODULE EIGHT   REFERENCES

The Buyer's Right – Consumer's Directory 1978 (Open University Press/ IOCU, 1978)
Advertising made simple (2nd Edition) F. Jenkins (W. H. Allen, 1977)
Annual Reports on Consumer policy in OECD member countries (OECD)
You and your rights: an A–Z guide to the law (Reader's Digest, 1980)
Consumers: know your rights J. Harries (Oyez, 1978)
Cases in Consumer Law H. Samuel (MacDonald & Evans, 1979)

Leaflets and booklets supplied by the Office of Fair Trading.

FOLLOW-UP ACTIVITIES

1. Find out about other National and International Organisations that can help the consumer.
2. Ascertain the advantages and disadvantages of the credit options available to consumers.
3. Obtain a hire purchase agreement and study it carefully.
4. Look at advertisements – attempt to discover the 'real' message – what is the advertiser really selling?
5. Collect as many labels or pictures of labels as possible. Consider how much useful information is provided.
6. Write a letter of complaint about faulty goods or a service which is not up to standard.
7. Examine guarantees and consider the meaning of statements.

FOOD

NOTE Before the study of this module it is advisable to revise basic nutrition. (*Refer to 'O' Level Cookery*)

It has been said that we are what we eat. Compare the starving children in Oxfam photographs with children in the UK. The basic reason for eating is to live – we become hungry and we want to eat. Primitive man had to eat what was available in order to survive, and there are people in the world who still have to do this. However, most people in the Western world are able to choose from a wide selection of foods, refuse to eat some foods and have food 'fads'. They should not suffer from undernutrition (when the body receives an insufficient amount of nutrients) but many people suffer from malnutrition (when the body receives the wrong amount or proportion of nutrients).

Malnutrition is occurring at a time when:
a) More is being written about food and health than possibly any other time.
b) Television advertisements emphasise the health value of foods.
c) Modern processing and quick transport make a wide variety of foods available.
d) Health food stores are in most towns.
e) Nutrition education is given in schools.
f) Advice is given to mothers in clinics and hospitals.
g) Food laws are much stricter.

CULTURE/TRADITION

The society in which people live influences what they eat – climate, type of local produce, religion, etc. Consider the food eaten in different countries and the regional food in the UK. When people taste food from other countries – from neighbours, on holiday, in restaurants, etc. they may add other types of food to their diet. Chinese and Indian dishes have become popular in the UK.

FOOD AT HOME

The type of food eaten and meal patterns can be:
a) Traditional 'sit-down' meals with several courses and varying amounts of nutrients.
b) Snack meals – nutritionally sound or mainly starch/sugar.
c) Little or no breakfast.
d) Entertaining other people and providing simple or elaborate meals.

FOOD EATEN OUT

Can vary in quality. Cost is usually high. It may be thought that a member of a family eating out is having a balanced meal and this could affect what is provided at home.
a) Subsidised meals provided by an authority, e.g. school meals, or a firm. Choice will vary but there is usually an alternative between a snack or a meal.
b) Use of luncheon vouchers or lunch allowance.
c) Use of pocket money depending on how much is available.
The choice of food in (a), (b) or (c) above may vary from a nutritionally balanced meal or snack to a choice of crisps/chips/cakes/biscuits, etc.
d) Social meals at restaurants – the choice tends to be in a meal pattern but may not necessarily be nutritionally sound.

LIKES AND DISLIKES

Likes and dislikes – are related to habits developed when young. Most foods are chosen because of likes and dislikes rather than nutritional balance.

Taste

a) *Sweet*
Children introduced to sweets and chocolate and other sweet foods at an early age develop a taste for 'sweetness' which often continues into adult

life. In the UK a hundred years ago, about 5 lb (2¼ kg) of sugar per head was eaten each year. Now an average of about 105 lb (47¼ kg) per head is eaten. In addition to the large variety of sweet foods available, sweetening in the form of sugar or sugar substitutes is added to a number of savoury foods, e.g. tinned soups and vegetables.

b) *Savoury*
Some of the liking for a savoury taste comes from additions of flavouring to make tasteless or 'bland' foods more acceptable, e.g. vinegar added to fish and chips; sauces added to pies and other food.

c) *Synthetic flavouring*
Synthetic flavours are added to make foods taste 'real', e.g. – to 'orange' drink containing no oranges (which may be preferred to the taste of orange juice and mistaken for it); in flavoured crisps.

Note: Monosodium glutamate is added to most packet and tinned savoury foods to *bring out* the flavour of the food. It is not a synthetic flavouring because it does not *add* flavour.

Appearance

a) *Colour*
Certain foods are expected to be a certain colour, e.g. bread is white or brown. Try putting some harmless blue vegetable colouring in bread dough and baking it, then serve it at a meal and observe the reaction. Experiments with processed peas – serving without and with added green colouring and no added flavouring – have resulted in comments about the better flavour of the coloured peas.
Brightness of colour is often associated with better flavour and freshness. This is not always a reliable guide.

b) *Texture*
People are showing a preference for soft foods which are easily eaten or crisp foods which do not require chewing but break easily. Food may be overcooked and lack flavour and nutritive value. There should be a balance of textures in a meal and 'chew' is needed to exercise the teeth and aid digestion.

COST

The cost of food is not related to the nutritive value it provides. Food may be cheap, e.g. liver, and provide more nutrients than other more expensive meat products. Some foods are very expensive, e.g. out-of-season straw-berries, prime cuts of meat, caviare, but they are still bought. Some foods contain a lot of 'bulk', e.g. fish cakes or fish fingers with a thick coating, or tinned meat and vegetables with little meat, and so are an expensive way to buy protein. However, as already considered, one of the main reasons for buying food is because of liking it. As income increases, usually the amount spent on food increases to obtain a wider variety – sometimes 'junk' foods with little nutritive or economic value. Spending more money on food does not mean that nutritional value will increase.

During the Second World War, when food was in very short supply, people in the UK were guided towards sound nutritional practices to try to maintain health and to avoid waste. With rationing, the amount of money which could be spent on food was limited. Sound nutrition had to be prac-tised – meat was 'stretched' with the addition of more vegetables; very little was removed from flour during milling and National flour and bread was eaten; the Oslo meal of cheese, wholemeal bread and raw vegetables was provided for school children; the shortage of sugar benefitted teeth.

At the present time, when food costs are rising and incomes are limited, it is necessary to consider nutritional needs, to find out how a balanced diet can be provided at a reasonable cost, and still supply enjoyable meals.

ADVERTISING (*Refer Module 8*)

Advertisements in magazines, and in particular on television, and labels and packaging, have a tremendous effect on the choice of food. There has to be truth in claims about food (*Refer to pp. 135–136*), but colour photography and presentation is so advanced that the pictures, together with the characters and jingles, 'sell' the food. People may not listen to, or look at, information about the ingredients or consider the value. Promotions in shops, displays and shelf-layouts are carefully planned to influence shoppers. Consider why sweets are placed at a low level at checkout points.

FOOD/HEALTH THEORIES

A number of sayings about food have been passed on from one generation to another, to encourage children to eat, e.g. 'An apple a day keeps the doctor away', or 'Fish is brain food'. (Without scientific evidence.)

Today there are a number of theories which have been developed relating food to health. It must be emphasised that there are differences of opinion about the truth of the theories.

Cholesterol and heart disease

It has been stated that high cholesterol levels in the blood increase the danger of heart disease. Foods which contain 'saturated' fat are thought to raise the blood cholesterol level, e.g. butter, cheese, cream, eggs, fat meat, dripping, lard. 'Polyunsaturated' fats are recommended, e.g. certain margarines and oils, and food with little fat – chicken, lean meat, fish, fruit and vegetables. The theory has resulted in some people, particularly men over the age of 45 years, changing their diet to cut down on saturated fats. Some medical authorities do not support the theory.

Dietary fibre and roughage

Dietary fibre is mainly obtained from bran in cereals, and cellulose and pectin in fruit and vegetables. It is sometimes referred to as roughage. Fibre is not a nutrient since it is not digested but it does assist the digestive process and can prevent constipation. When cereals are processed, e.g. wheat into white flour, much of the bran is removed and little dietary fibre is available. If insufficient fruit and vegetables are eaten or if they are peeled and overcooked, little fibre will be added to the diet. It has been suggested by some nutritionists that extra dietary fibre in the form of bran should be added to food or that wholemeal or 'hibran' bread should be eaten. Other experts consider that a balanced diet should contain sufficient dietary fibre or roughage, and that adding more might not be beneficial.

Obesity and slimming

It has been stated that between the months of February and July one in three women in the UK, and a number of men, are on some form of diet in preparation for holidays and the wearing of summer clothes. Obesity, the state of being over-weight, often runs in families because of the amount and type of food eaten. Children in such families develop the habit of overeating or a liking for foods which promote fatness. Except for people with certain illnesses, e.g. hormone imbalance, most fat people eat the wrong amount or type of food. Extra weight which is carried by fat people is thought to be a contributory factor to a number of health problems including heart disease.

Practically every week magazines publish slimming diets and there are a number of slimming clubs and health farms. Diets are based on a reduction of the amount/type of food eaten, usually a reduction of carbohydrates and fats. While most people would benefit from some reduction in certain foods, cutting down the intake of food drastically is not advisable. People in poor health should not diet except by medical advice. Anyone considering a strict diet should ask the doctor's opinion. Anorexia Nervosa is a deficiency disease in which people starve themselves to become thin. It has resulted in severe illness and death. (*Refer Module 6*)

If suitable food is eaten in the right proportion, good health should be maintained and slimming should not be necessary.

Vitamins and minerals

The importance of vitamins and minerals in maintaining health is often stressed in articles on nutrition and in advertisements. This has led many people to think that if they take extra supplies they will be healthy. Tablets and capsules are available which contain synthetic vitamins and minerals. If these are taken in small doses they may contribute a little to a healthy diet but in large amounts they could cause harm. The advice of a doctor should be obtained. A balanced diet should provide all the vitamins and minerals required except during and after an illness when they will be prescribed if necessary.

FOOD ADDITIVES

An examination of the ingredients written in small print on food packets and cans will often show a list of chemicals as well as food ingredients. A food additive is a chemical substance added to food that is not naturally present in the food.
Included are:
a) *Preservatives*
   To prevent decay and increase shelf life,
   e.g. – Sodium and potassium nitrites in tinned meats.
         Sodium and calcium compounds in baked products.
         Antioxidants in packet soups, dried potato, some fats and oils.
b) *Emulsifiers*
   To provide stable emulsions, i.e. which will not separate out, e.g. glycerol monostearate (GMS) in ice-cream, salad creams, margarines.
c) *Anti-caking agents*
   To keep dry ingredients free flowing, e.g. silicates added to dry mixes.

d) *Flavourings*
   1. To enhance natural flavour – monosodium glutamate in savoury canned and packet foods.
   2. To provide flavours artificially – e.g. ethyl acetate for apple, peach, pear and strawberry flavours.
   3. To add sweetness – sugar or artificial sweeteners, e.g. sorbitol, saccharine, are added to a number of foods.

e) *Colourings*
   1. To replace colours lost in processing, e.g. tinned vegetables.
   2. To imitate the 'real' food, e.g. in 'fruit' drinks, sweets or desserts which do not contain fruit.

f) *Nutrients*
   To provide added nutritive value or to replace nutrients lost by processing, e.g. calcium, iron, vitamins of the B group added to bread.
   Vitamin C added to dried potato, fruit drinks.
   Vegetable protein (TVP) to 'extend' meat in tinned and packaged meat products.

g) *Fluoride*
   Added to some water supplies as a prevention against tooth decay.

Note: HERBICIDES. When soil and crops are sprayed with chemicals to kill pests and weeds, the food crops may become contaminated. This is particularly dangerous in fruit and vegetables which are eaten raw and may not have been washed.

Pollution by chemicals from industry is also possible. (*Refer Module 6*)

FOOD LEGISLATION IN UK

Note: It is only possible to give basic information because of the vast amount of legislation.

The law requires:
1. *No dishonesty in trading*
   Food must be the type, weight and quality stated.
2. *Food should be hygienic*
   Ingredients should be pure.
   Production, distribution, storage and handling must be carried out subject to hygiene regulations.
3. *Animals must be killed in the most hygienic and humane manner*
   There are rules for abattoirs, poultry keepers, etc.

4. *Substitute ingredients are not allowed*
Unless this is permitted by law and indicated on the label.

5. *Labelling must be correct*
Information must be true and all ingredients must be indicated. Some may be grouped, e.g. mixed herbs. Water content is not usually required. Ingredients (including additives) should be printed in descending weight order. The size of lettering and the position of certain information on labels is stipulated.

6. *Date marking is required for certain foods*
Date marking must be related to the 'total life' of the food, which is defined as being 'the length of time a food remains acceptable for consumption'. Foods are divided into categories according to type. Manufacturers have to print a 'sell by' date which must be less than 'total life' to allow storage in the home before consumption.

7. *No false and misleading claims*
It should not be stated, if it is not true, that food contains certain nutrients; is of value to health; is an aid to slimming, etc.

8. *Information about origin should be given*
The name of the manufacturer, packer, importer or seller must be included.

WORLD RESOURCES OF FOOD

While there is an over-abundance of food for people in the West, in other parts of the world people are dying because of a lack of food and water. It has been said that there is plenty of food in the world but that it is not distributed efficiently, in spite of technological advances in food production and processing and the increased speed of travel.

Attempts which have been made to improve food production include:

1. The wider use of fertilisers and pesticides.
2. Better irrigation or drainage.
3. Co-operation with small farmers in remote areas to try to develop more efficient cultivation.
4. The use of agricultural land to raise crops and not to graze animals.
5. The production of novel protein foods from cheap, plentiful vegetable sources. Soya beans, sometimes with added ground nuts and field nuts, are already used to produce textured vegetable protein (TVP) which can be manufactured to resemble minced meat or chunks of meat and fish. It is

used to mix with meat or fish as an 'extender' or as a substitute. Experiments are being made with other vegetables.

6. Battery farming, e.g. for the production of eggs and poultry.

7. Fish farming. The use of whole fish and fish minces is capable of much wider development.

Experiments are being made to try to produce food from the most unlikely materials – sugar from sawdust; protein from wool, yeasts, fungi, algae, bacteria. It is to be hoped that soon all the people of the world will have an adequate supply of food which is suitable for their needs.

PROVIDING A BALANCED DIET

1. A knowledge of nutrition.

2. An appreciation of the nutritional needs of individuals in the family and how to combine and provide for these needs in family meals.

3. Choosing, storing, preparing, cooking and serving food to preserve nutrients.

4. Providing 'food' as well as nutrients. People choose, eat and enjoy food, not nutrients. As well as providing for nutritional needs, it is necessary to consider likes and dislikes (provided that these are not excessive), taste, appearance, texture.

5. Food and social occasions. Meals are often used as an occasion to entertain friends and relatives. This may be at a festival like Christmas, at a wedding, at a birthday party, a meal out in a restaurant or morning coffee. These are opportunites to combine food with pleasure and to learn more about the enjoyment of food.

6. Children should be guided to enjoy food which is nutritionally sound and to appreciate the pleasure of eating good food.

MODULE NINE   REFERENCES

'O' Level Cookery Abbey and MacDonald (Methuen Educational)
The Wholefood Book G. Seddon /J. Burrow (Mitchell Beazley)
In Search of Food D. and R. Mabey (Macdonald & Jane's)
Food Labelling Guide (Food Manufacturers Federation)
Food Standards Committee Report on Food Labelling (HMSO)
Articles on food and nutrition

FOLLOW-UP ACTIVITIES

1. Examine a selection of labels and information packaging. Consider the wording and illustrations. List the ingredients and try to identify their use.
2. Investigate the use of novel proteins. Cook and serve foods containing the proteins. Compare the cost, convenience of cooking and serving, and taste, with similar foods containing all meat.
3. Prepare a selection of foods for tasting. Include some sweet and some savoury foods, some 'real' and some synthetic foods, e.g. orange juice, and various textures. Arrange a 'blindfold' test by a panel of people to consider identification of foods, likes and dislikes, etc.
4. Compare traditional foods of the UK with those from other countries.
5. Collect information about food shortages in the world.
6. Examine some published slimming diets and work out the nutritional value and the possible deficiencies in the diet. Consider the cost.

CLOTHING

The term 'clothing' means 'covering for the human body'. It is usual to include accessories, e.g. shoes, bags, belts, scarves and jewellery in this term. The first clothes were the skins of animals; the bones and teeth were used as fastenings and jewellery. The styles for men and women were similar, e.g. tunic, cape, moccasins or boots. The range of clothing increased with the techniques of spinning, weaving and dyeing fibres and yarns.

FUNCTIONS

Clothing is worn to keep the body:
a) *warm* – Clothing can be made from textiles which are textured, or made from hair, fur or wool. These materials have the property to trap pockets of air and so the body is kept warm. Layers of thin clothing have the same effect.
b) *cool* – Body heat is lost by sweating so clothes made from textiles that absorb sweat and dry quickly (e.g. cotton, linen) are ideal for wearing in hot climates.
c) *dry* – The ability to resist water penetration is based on the production of a fabric with a close weave with a filling or coating, e.g. PVC or moisture-proof cotton.

Clothing is also worn:
d) *to give protection*, e.g. in industry or sports.
e) *to look attractive* – This is one of the main reasons why people choose clothes.
f) *to indicate group membership*, e.g. occupation.
g) *for fashion*

General considerations about clothing
a) Needs of individual members of the family: age, sex, work, leisure, health, personal attributes (e.g. colouring, height, build).
b) Money available – cash or credit.
c) Time available for making or buying.
d) Laundry facilities available, e.g. automatic washing machine, launderette, dry cleaners.
e) Season of the year – warm clothes are usually needed in the winter.
f) Shopping facilities available, e.g. department store, boutique, chain store, market, shoe shops, mail order catalogue.
g) Individual skills – dressmaking, tailoring, designing, repairing.
h) Present wardrobe to be assessed as needs can change.

Choice of individual garments – occasion, fashion, colour, size, fabric, cost, ease of laundering, durability.

FAMILY NEEDS AND GUIDELINES

Needs of individuals in a family – vary considerably.
Baby   Toddler   Boys and girls up to 13 years
Adolescents   Women   Men
Elderly people

Baby
(*Refer to Module 3 for details of layette*)

Toddler

This is a period of rapid growth and activity. Clothing is needed which does not hinder movement or restrict growth. Choice is influenced by use: day-wear, nightwear, outdoor, special occasions.

Guidelines: clothing needs to:
a) have simple fastenings to help toddler in learning to dress and undress;
b) be durable;
c) be functional;
d) be easy to launder;
e) look attractive;
f) have allowance for growth, e.g. tucks, double hems, long straps.

Clothing suggestions

Daywear	*Nightwear*	*Outdoor wear*	*Special occasions*
Dungarees, socks, skirt, tights, jumpers, blouses/shirts, playsuits, protective clothing for play.	Nightdresses, pyjamas (**N.B.** flame-resistant finish).	Rainwear, summer/winter coat, duffle coat, anorak, all-in-one suit, blazer for summer, headwear, mittens.	Trouser suit, party dress.

Underwear
Vests, trainer pants.

Boys and girls aged 6–12 years

During this stage boys and girls are growing rapidly. They should be able to dress and undress themselves by the time they start school. Some schools require uniform. *All* clothing worn in school should be clearly marked with the child's name. At this stage some children start to be aware of fashion.

Guidelines
a) Until the primary school child is really competent at dressing and undressing, ensure fastenings are easy.
b) When children are out in poor light, luminous armbands or patches should be attached to outdoor clothing so that they can be seen easily by motorists.
c) Unless a uniform is required, the guidelines for the toddler can also be followed.

Clothing suggestions

Daywear		Nightwear	Outdoor wear	Special occasions
School Uniform (if specified), skirts, cardigans/tops/ jumpers, trousers, jeans, dresses, blouses/shirts, protective	clothing for practical classes PE kit, tights, socks *Leisure* Similar to daywear, tracksuit, sportswear.	Nightdresses, pyjamas (N.B.flame- resistant finish).	Uniform (if specified), duffle coat, winter coat, summer coat, anorak, mackintosh, blazer.	Confirmation, bridesmaid, page outfit, long dress, trouser suit, dresses (long or short).

Underwear
Pants, vests, underskirts. Some girls may need a bra towards the end of this age range.

Adolescents

This is a period of rapid growth and development and great activity. Adolescents may be in two categories:
a) Those still at school who may be required to wear a uniform.
b) Those working who may also need a 'uniform', e.g. nurse, armed services.
   Adolescents require clothes for leisure.

Guidelines and suggestions
a) Choose according to style of living, e.g. school, work, leisure. Some clothes are multi-purpose and are suitable for a variety of occasions.
b) Ease of laundering – look at care labels. (*Refer Book 2 – The Home*)
c) Take into account figure type and personal colouring so that an attractive appearance results.
d) Be aware of fashion trends.
e) Use personal skills to make items of clothing to save expense.

Women

Women may be at home or working, or may be expectant or nursing a baby. Most women are fashion conscious.

Guidelines and suggestions
a) Choose according to style of living.
b) Suggestions for clothing during pregnancy are made in Module 2.
c) Figure type and personal colouring should be taken into account.
d) A clothing allowance from the family budget is available for some women. Money can be saved by making clothes.
e) A uniform (nursing, police), protective clothing. A clothing allowance is paid by some employers.

Men

Needs are influenced by occupation, the amount of leisure time available, income and interest in clothing. It is not unusual for the women in the family to purchase a significant number of items of clothing for the men. Most men tend to have a basic wardrobe of suits and separates and a variety of accessories. There may be an awareness of fashion trends.

Guidelines and suggestions
a) Choose according to style of living. A uniform or overalls or an allowance may be available depending on the place of employment.
b) Hobbies or interests may influence clothing for leisure.
c) Figure type and personal colouring should be taken into account.

Elderly people

The majority of elderly people are no longer in full-time employment so their needs are modified (*Refer Module 5*).

Guidelines and suggestions
a) Clothing is influenced by hobbies and interests.
b) Choose according to figure type and personal colouring (these can change with age).
c) Many experience difficulty in maintaining body temperature especially in winter; warm underwear and weather-proof outer garments are advisable.
d) On dark evenings it is advisable to wear something light-coloured to be visible to motorists.

Body measurements

Whether an individual chooses to make or buy clothing it is important to be able to identify personal size.

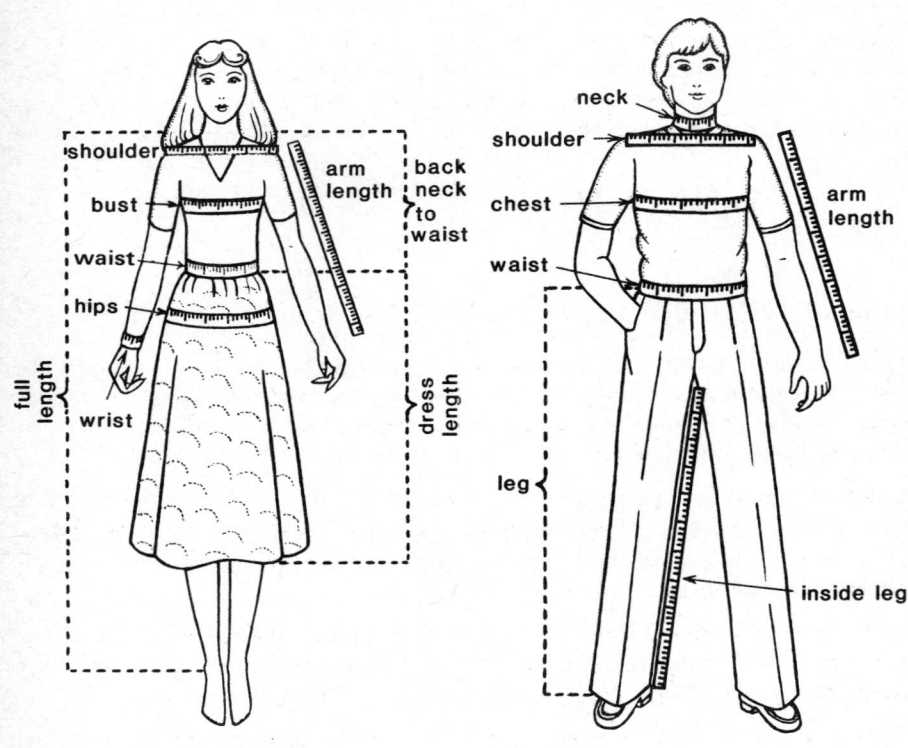

Body measurements can vary so it is advisable to check frequently, especially during childhood and adolescence or if weight loss or gain during adulthood. If clothes are made at home, it is advisable to adapt a basic pattern to body measurements and use this to adjust other patterns.

Foundation garments

For many women and girls the correct fitting of clothes depends upon the choice and fit of foundation garments.

Bra

When choosing a bra it should be the correct size, fit correctly and be comfortable. Bra sizes are in several cup sizes, e.g.

> A (small)   B (medium)   C (large)

Bust size – under arm measurement, above the bust.

Cup size – fullest part of the bust.

2·5 cm larger than bra size – cup A

2·5–5 cm larger than bra size – cup B

5–7·5 cm larger than bra size – cup C

Girdle

A number of women need the support provided by a well-fitting girdle or similar garment.

Colour, texture, line, cut and fit

It has been stated that one of the reasons for wearing clothes is to make the body look attractive. Colour, texture, style, line, cut and fit can all contribute. But an individual needs to be aware of what is personally suitable. This depends on the size, proportion and colouring of the individual.

Colour is important in clothing. People's sense of colour varies. Colour choice should be related to personal colouring. Colours can be used to create effects, e.g. dark colours appear to reduce size, bright and light colours appear to increase size.

Fabric patterns should relate to garment style and body shape, e.g. large patterns may not be suitable. Horizontal stripes can make the wearer look shorter and fatter. Vertical stripes can achieve the opposite effect.

Texture can be rough, smooth, shiny, soft, etc. This should relate to style.

Style refers to cut and involves variations in shape, length, type of sleeve, neckline, etc. This used to change with fashion and people would follow each style as it was produced, e.g. 'crinoline', 'new look', 'mini', 'flared' or 'drain pipe' trousers. Nowdays there is much more freedom and a mixture of styles are worn by people of all ages and sexes.

Clothing choice

Choosing clothing is very personal but it is a matter of being able to:

a) identify needs and preferences;

b) recognise which styles, textures, colours, fashions accentuate the good features;

c) recognise figure limitations.

When making decisions about personal clothing and for family members the question arises – to make or buy?

Factors affecting this decision include:

a) individual skills in dressmaking, tailoring, knitting, crochet;

b) time available;

c) money available – cash or credit.

There are certain advantages in making clothes if one has the necessary skills:

a) money can be saved as off-the-peg clothing can be expensive;

b) remnants can be bought cheaply;

c) individuality can be achieved in style; design; fit; fabric and colour.

If the decision is taken to purchase clothing, the following points should be considered:

a) style;

b) fabric and colour;

c) size – measurements can vary from one manufacturer to another;

d) fitting – depends on body proportions;

e) details/trimmings – belts, collars, buttons, top stitching;

f) construction – seams, lining, finishing, hems.

g) care – can garment be washed or is dry cleaning required?

Final considerations – price, suitability for occasion, alterations required.

FOOTWEAR

The needs of family members vary but there are basic rules about footwear which must be followed to ensure healthy feet.

a) Permanent damage or deformation can result if the wrong footwear is worn.

b) It is unwise to buy poor quality shoes since they may damage the feet by rubbing, pinching, weakening the arch. Quality is not always related to price since expensive shoes are not necessarily well-constructed.

c) Second-hand footwear should *not* be worn. The shape of the foot is moulded into the footwear during wear and will be different for each individual. Infections, e.g. verrucas, may be transmitted.

d) Consider: size; fitting (length and width); height of heel; material (upper and sole); style.
e) Tights and socks should be the correct size and changed daily. **N.B.** Some people are allergic to nylon.
f) Slippers must fit securely and be the correct size. They do not always provide the necessary support.
g) Wellingtons should only be worn for short periods because:
   (i) little support is provided;
   (ii) they are not porous and make feet perspire and become cold. Always wear with socks.
h) Boots may be for protection against weather or 'fashion' boots. When choosing, be aware of the difference. Wearing boots made from synthetic fabrics for long periods can be harmful.

NEEDS OF FAMILY MEMBERS

Baby

Shoes are generally unnecessary until the walking stage – knitted or crocheted bootees are sufficient to keep the feet warm. Footwear is necessary at the crawling stage to protect the feet.

Toddler

At the early walking stage it is vital to choose footwear carefully because the full weight of the body is carried by the feet. The toddler should be taken to a reputable shop where feet should be measured accurately on a gauge. Size and fitting should be checked every 3 months. Until the child has achieved balance, wellingtons are not advisable (see previous notes).

School children

There may be regulations for school wear. Gym shoes should not be worn for long periods since they do not allow feet to breathe. It is advisable to take an extra pair of shoes to school in wet weather so that wet shoes are not worn all day.

Adolescents

If still at school, regulations may apply. Fashion consciousness develops and some footwear fashions can cause deformities. A special type of footwear may be needed for some jobs (nurses, factory workers). Employers give advice and often supply footwear or provide an allowance.

Adults

Choice is influenced by style of living. Footwear is expensive so colours and styles should be chosen which are multi-purpose, if possible, and contrast/harmonise with clothing and other accessories.

Elderly people

Footwear should be well fitting, comfortable and give the correct support. A number of accidents are caused by wearing loose fitting shoes or slippers.

ACCESSORIES

When selecting items of clothing, decisions also need to be made about accessories. These are used to contrast or harmonise with outfits, e.g. scarves, belts, bags, ties, jewellery.

DAY-TO-DAY CARE OF CLOTHES, SHOES AND ACCESSORIES

a) Hang clothes outside storage area to air for a few hours or overnight before putting away.
b) Use a clothes brush to remove dust, etc.
c) Use protective clothing for cleaning tasks.
d) Remove stains as soon as possible.
e) Clean shoes regularly – check if repairs necessary.
f) Clean out handbags regularly.
g) Never store wet clothing – hang up in a suitable place to dry.
h) Allow wet footwear to dry out at room temperature – stuff with newspaper to maintain shape.
i) Empty pockets, close fastenings to ensure shape of garments is maintained.
j) Carry out repairs when necessary.
k) Perspiration not only has odour, it will rot clothes so they should be washed/dry cleaned frequently.

STORAGE

Clothes need careful storage to keep them in good condition. Maintenance and laundering (*Refer Book 2 – The Home*). Storage depends on facilities in the home.

a) Height of cupboard/wardrobe should be such that hems do not touch floor or base.
b) Depth of cupboard/wardrobe should be sufficient to allow clothing to hang without touching cupboard/wardrobe back or door.
c) Do not attempt to fit more clothes into the storage space than it is designed to take – unnecessary creasing will result.
d) Skirts and trousers should be hung on special hangers.
e) Underwear, sweaters, scarves, gloves can be stored in drawers. Ties – in racks or over piece of expanding curtain wire fixed to cupboard door.
f) Blouses/shirts stay uncreased if put on to coat hangers after ironing.
g) Footwear and handbags may be stored on shelves fitted inside wardrobe/cupboard or in base of wardrobe/cupboard.
h) Precautions should be taken to prevent moth/mildew damage.

MODULE TEN REFERENCES

Complete Guide to Sewing (Readers Digest Assoc., 1978)
Needlework Rosalie P. Giles (Methuen Educational, 1972)
Fashion Journals

FOLLOW-UP ACTIVITIES

1. Visit a library or a museum and find out about clothing in past centuries. Choose a garment, e.g. blouse/shirt, and trace how it evolved into its present form.
2. Design a suitable outfit for a special occasion.
3. Make a simple garment for a toddler or a bag for yourself from a remnant of fabric. Compare the price of a similar ready-made article in different shops.
4. Visit a market, a department store and a boutique and compare the prices and quality of a skirt/pair of trousers.
5. Examine the clothes you have and carry out any necessary maintenance. Consider how you could update one of your garments. Draw a sketch and explain how this could be achieved.

OBJECTIVES

MODULE ONE   IDENTIFICATION OF THE FAMILY

Objectives   After this module you should be able to:
1. Identify types of families.
2. List the functions of families.

MODULE TWO   BABY AND CHILD DEVELOPMENT

Objectives   After this module you should be able to:
1. Explain how conception occurs.
2. Recognise the signs of pregnancy.
3. Be aware of different methods of contraception.
4. Explain the stages of foetal growth during pregnancy.
5. Appreciate the importance of sound antenatal care to the mother and her unborn child.
6. State how a baby is born.
7. Appreciate the importance of postnatal care.
8. Be aware of the developmental processes of a pre-school child.
9. Describe the father's role in pregnancy and child development.

MODULE THREE   BABY AND CHILD CARE

Objectives   After this module you should be able to:
1. Describe the role of the parents in baby and child care.
2. List the factors affecting the choice of layette and equipment.
3. List the advantages and disadvantages of breast and bottle feeding.
4. Describe the procedures for a) bathing, b) nappy changing.

5. Appreciate the importance of safety.
6. Consider
   a) the safety aspect of toys,
   b) the educational aspect of toys.
7. Examine the community provision available to the family.

MODULE FOUR   CHILDHOOD TO ADULTHOOD

Objectives   After this module you should be able to:
1. State what is meant by the terms 'puberty'; 'adolescence'.
2. Consider development up to the age of puberty.
3. List the main stages in the physical and sexual development of adolescents.
4. Consider the intellectual, emotional and social development of adolescents.

MODULE FIVE   THE ELDERLY

Objectives   After this module you should be able to:
1. List the needs of the elderly.
2. Identify the characteristics of the ageing process in the human body.
3. State the problems associated with retirement.
4. Recognise the effect on family life of an elderly relative living in the family home.
5. Be aware of community provision available for the elderly.

MODULE SIX   HEALTH

Objectives   After this module you should be able to:
1. Describe the development of health care in Great Britain and identify some of the main stages in the development.
2. Explain the importance of a positive approach to health for physical and mental well-being.
3. Identify the causes of infection.
4. State the main steps to be taken to prevent disease.
5. Identify some health hazards.
6. Explain the importance of sound nutritional practices.
7. Define the term 'drugs' and state the dangers involved in their abuse.

8. List the causes of accidents and be aware of a positive approach to safety.
9. Appreciate the need for a knowledge of first aid.
10. Explain the structure of the National Health Service and state the main provisions of the Service.
11. Identify the personal care which is necessary to try to ensure body health and efficient functioning.
12. Identify the health concerns of the family.
13. Explain the need for community health provisions and list the main areas.

MODULE SEVEN   FINANCE

Objectives   After this module you should be able to:
1. Define the terms concerned with the payment of wages/salary.
2. Consider the income and expenditure of the country.
3. Explain the assessment and collection of:
   a) income tax, b) rates.
4. Define the terms concerned with money management.
5. List the areas of income and expenditure and explain the importance of budgeting.
6. State the reasons for saving or investing and outline the types of saving/ investment which are available.
7. Consider the functions of banks.
   a) outline the services which a bank offers,
   b) explain how to use bank accounts.
8. Define the terms concerned with insurance.
9. Consider the insurance/assurance which is necessary.
10. List the main areas of community provision and explain the process of obtaining assistance.

MODULE EIGHT   THE CONSUMER

Objectives   After this module you should be able to:
1. Define the word 'consumer'.
2. Give a brief account of the historical development of the consumer movement in the United Kingdom.
3. Be aware of the rights and obligations of the consumer under the law.

4. List and describe the shops and shopping facilities available to the consumer.
5. Appreciate the influence of advertising in everyday life.
6. Recall the credit facilities available to the consumer.
7. Describe the types of labels and explain their functions.
8. State the procedure for making a complaint.
9. Summarise the effect of EEC membership on the consumer.

MODULE NINE   FOOD

Objectives   After this module you should be able to:
1. Explain the reasons for choosing and eating food.
2. Consider food habits and their effect on the food eaten, and standards of nutrition and health.
3. Define the term 'food additive' and consider the types of additive in use.
4. Explain what novel proteins are and give examples of their use.
5. State some of the theories about food and health and consider arguments for and against the theories.
6. Consider the dangers of obesity and slimming.
7. Consider food legislation and explain how this influences food production and advertising.
8. Be aware of world food problems.

MODULE TEN   CLOTHING

Objectives   After this module you should be able to:
1. Identify the clothing needs of individual family members.
2. State the reasons why clothes are worn.
3. Determine your personal measurements.
4. Appreciate the importance of colour, line, texture and style when choosing clothing.
5. List the points to note when buying articles of clothing.
6. State the care procedure for garments and accessories.
7. Be aware of the influence of fashion.

CONCLUSION

The contents of this book give an indication of the breadth and depth of matters concerned with the family. As already stated, the family is a unit composed of individuals who may range from a baby to an elderly person. There are general family concerns involving all family members who can contribute, but individuals need relationships within their own age groups. There is also a need for understanding, tolerance and caring between different age groups. To achieve understanding, knowledge about the requirements at different stages of life is necessary. A study of the aspects of Home Economics provided in this book should prove beneficial.

INDEX